ISBN 0-9667295-0-1
Library of Congress Catalog Card Number: 98-92140

CONTENTS:

Cholesterol Drug Helps Save Lives
-Tim Friend, USA TODAY, Nov. 17, 1994

BYPASSING HEART SURGERY, CHANGES IN DIET DO SLOW OR REVERSE HEART DISEASE

Patient Calls Ornish Program "Miraculous" Initial Study Was Greeted by Skepticism
-Tim Friend, USA TODAY, Sept. 20, 1995

Study finds medical care influenced by geography
- Steven Findlay USA TODAY Oct 15, 1997

Comment: *If you cannot get medical treatment you deserve in the place you live,* ***prevention may be the best option.*** *-Dr. Pai*

Businesses leery of health care quality
-Steven Findlay, USA TODAY

DOCTORS FAIL TO FULLY TREAT HEART DISEASE
Tim Friend, USA TODAY

American Heart Association President Dr. Sidney Smith criticized physicians at the AHA's scientific sessions in Anaheim, California in Nov 1995, for not offering well-established treatments.

Experts say **doctors don't make patients reduce their risk factors. Patients often won't follow advice, and insurance won't pay** for simple programs to help patients change behavior *(and thus modify cardiac risk factors.)*

Cholesterol pill may help the healthy
-Rita Rubin USA TODAY May 27, 1998

Millions Not Taking Life-Saving Drug, Research Reveals "It's A Sad Commentary"

-Diana K. Sugg The Sun, Baltimore, MD, April 19, 1998

Medicine Can Lower Cholesterol and Prevent Heart Attacks

Broader Benefit Found In Drug For Cholesterol

-Gina Kolata, N.Y. Times, May, 27 1998)

Many doctors themselves who heard about the benefits of Lovastatin study have already begun taking Lovastatin or another newer cholesterol lowering statin. **Among doctors the question is not whether** you are taking a (cholesterol lowering) statin or not, **but which statin are you taking.**

A New Generation Of Tests To Find Heart Trouble Early.

-Gina Kolata, The New York Times, Nov. 26, 1995

Women More Likely to Die After Bypass

-Rita Rubin USA TODAY July 30, 1998

(Recent studies show no gender difference in deaths after bypass)

Heart Disease Gap Widens Between Blacks, Whites

-Andrea Stone USA TODAY page 3A Nov 13, 1998

(Death Rate Bl male 1.5 x WH male, BL fm 2 x WH fm)

(Calculated from CDC figures)

3

FINDINGS ON CORONARY ARTERY DISEASE
by N.M. Pai, M.D.

I have collected data on coronary artery disease for the last several years, but in the last five years there has been groundbreaking research on prevention and reversal of heart disease, most of which emphasizes dietary and lifestyle modification, cholesterol-lowering drugs and a combination of vitamins and other antioxidants.

About 25 years ago I coined the **term Atherolysis™ to designate my program for the prevention and reversal of atherosclerosis.** Today this process involves the use of a **combination of drugs, modification of diet and lifestyle,** and strict timing of drug administration to avoid adverse drug interactions (for example, avoiding concomitant use of erythromycin and some cholesterol-lowering statins). Though a goal of anatomical changes to restore the lumen of the coronary artery is desired, favorable physiological changes occur with minimal anatomic (i.e., reversal of blockages) changes – **mostly by plaque stabilization – thus preventing plaque**

4

rupture, which causes heart attacks. Restoration of Endothelial function helps the inner lining of the arteries (intima) to function normally.

The epidemic of cardiac arrests due to cardiovascular disease has turned our emergency rooms into "cardiac massage parlors." **350,000 heart attack victims will die this year before they receive any treatment at all.**

There has been overwhelming evidence for **prevention and reversal** of **heart disease** at the **American College of Cardiology** Annual Meeting at Anaheim, California, in March 1997; the **International Conference on Preventive Cardiology** at Montreal, Canada, in July 1997, and the **American Heart Association** Meeting at Orlando, Florida, in November 1997.

In our democracy we emphasize life, liberty, **and the pursuit of happiness, but never before has the pursuit of happiness been a major threat to life and liberty.**

According to professor Kelly Brownell of Yale University, **Americans have an unprecedented access to a poor diet,** to **high calo-**

rie foods that are **widely available, low in cost, heavily promoted** and **taste good**. These ingredients produce a **predictable, un-derstandable and inevitable consequence – an epidemic of diet related diseases.**

While blood cholesterol and dietary satu-rated fat may be among the most prominent coronary risk factors, a majority of people who are concerned about coronary disease are focused on these and ignore other im-portant risk factors.

Articles published in the Aug, 11 1997, is-sue of *Newsweek* and the August 4, 1997, issue of *Time magazine* alluded to a variety of innovative ways the risk factors may be controlled. The November/December, 1997 issue of *Health* carried an article titled, ***"Could You Catch A Heart Attack?"*** The February, 1998 issue of *Harvard Men's Health Watch* featured an article titled ***"Is Atherosclerosis an Infectious Disease?"***

In medicine, most of the information travels at the speed of light, but the information from research to public health travels at the speed of an Amish buggy (a horse-drawn carriage), which is – to say the least – a nagging problem. Millions of lives are lost even while medical knowledge is being transferred from research to public health. The purpose of this **book is to raise public awareness** and encourage people to make choices which most people never knew they had.

Listed herein are the new research findings, coupled with a few old ones. All the points raised are from standard textbooks, journals and medical newsletters. The information which people get from newspapers, news magazines and TV has also been analyzed.

While writing this book I have **attempted** to **minimize the technical terminology** and at the same time **avoid being overtly simplistic.**

As different people react differently to the same drugs, **patients and their doctors should decide as to what type of therapy is best suited for the patient.**

A detailed bibliography is out of scope for this (pocket-size) book, but specific references are offered where attribution is most appropriate. Some of the language in this book may sound strong or unpleasant, but so is the message of coronary artery disease and cardiac death. Certain explanations

7

have been provided to simplify complicated medical studies. If you have any questions, you can ask your doctor to answer them.

This book is not intended to be a self-medication guide, as self-medication could be fatal or cause major irreversible complications. Some important non-cardiac medical information (cancer, drug interactions, sleep deprivation, etc.) has also been added. Any reference to **risk** in this book refers to **cardiovascular risk** unless stated otherwise.

This book may also be useful to medical students and health care providers to concentrate on prevention.

Medical knowledge changes rapidly, but many drugs and treatments I have discussed in this book have been shown to save lives. So for the time being this book is current.

This book was inspired by my father, the late Professor M. P. Pai, M.S., F.R.C.S., F.A.C.S., F.A.M.S., an internationally-known professor of surgery who always professed excellence in medical care and compassion, understanding and caring for patients.

8

That which can be foreseen can be prevented.
—William J. Mayo, M.D.

WHAT DO YOU REALLY KNOW ABOUT HEART DISEASE?

Check your Heart Facts before and after reading this book!

Before proceeding further, try to answer the following questions to test your knowledge about heart disease. After you have finished reading the book, come back to page 10 and review these questions. *(The answers are on pages 102-103 of the book.)*

HEART DISEASE KNOWLEDGE QUIZ...

1. Cardiovascular disease kills more Americans than cancer, AIDS, all types of accidents, suicides and homicides combined.

TRUE / FALSE

2. Heart Disease is the No. 1 killer of Americans can women.

TRUE / FALSE

3. Heart Disease kills more women than men.

TRUE / FALSE

4. The process of atherosclerosis (fatty buildup within the arteries) starts as early as age two years.

TRUE / FALSE

5. Homocysteine is responsible for about ten percent of all cardiovascular deaths.

TRUE / FALSE

6. Chlamydia – a sexually-transmitted disease – may cause coronary artery disease.

TRUE / FALSE

7. Gingivitis (periodontal gum disease) may contribute to heart disease.

TRUE / FALSE

8. Moderate alcoholic beverage intake can decrease the risk of heart disease.

TRUE / FALSE

9. Beer bingeing is associated with increased heart disease.

TRUE / FALSE

10. There are adequate preventive cardiology services to handle the epidemic of heart disease.

TRUE / FALSE

11. Cholesterol lowering statins have more benefits than just lowering cholesterol.

TRUE / FALSE

12. A person with a normal EKG, echocardiogram and stress test can still have a heart attack without warning.

TRUE / FALSE

13. Lowering cholesterol levels even in normal people protect against cardiovascular disease.

TRUE / FALSE

14. Saturated fat content of the food is more important than the cholesterol content in raising blood cholesterol.

TRUE / FALSE

Answers page 102-103

11

PLEASE CONSIDER THE FOLLOWING:

1. Heart disease is the most common cause of death in the United States, Canada, United Kingdom, Europe, Russia, and China.

2. **One million Americans die every year; 2,700 die every day from cardiovascular disease.**

3. Annual deaths from lung cancer, 160,400; colorectal cancer, 54,900; breast cancer 44,190; prostate cancer, 41,800: AIDS, 32,655: motor vehicle accidents, 43,449: other accidents, 50,425: suicides, 30,862: and homicides, 20,738.

4. **30% of all heart attack patients have no known risk factors**

5. 40% of all deaths in the U.S. are direct result of cardiac and vascular diseases. More than **6 million people are living with coronary artery disease.**

6. **Heart disease is the number-one killer of American women.**

7. Cardiovascular disease **kills more women (51.9%) than men (48.1%).**

8. More women die from heart disease than from cancer.

9. Cardiovascular disease kills eleven times more women **than breast cancer.**

10. Cardiovascular disease **kills more** women than **all forms of cancer, chronic lung disease, pneumonia, diabetes, accidents and AIDS combined.**

11. 250,000 deaths due to coronary artery disease in the U.S. occur **within one hour** of the onset of symptoms.

12. 75,000 patients die instantly from heart disease. (Some patients are found dead several hours later like Gov. Lawton Chiles of Fl.)

13. One American **dies of heart disease every thirty seconds and one every minute from heart attack.**

14. Post-mortem on 19-year-old U.S. **soldiers** in Korea have **shown fatty deposits in the arteries.** Similar **fatty deposits have** been seen in the arteries of girls as young as 15 during autopsies of 364 women between **the ages of 15 and 34** who died from accidents, murder or suicide. (*Tufts University Health & Nutrition Letter, April, 1997*)

Bogalusa Heart Study – fatty streaks in children 2 to 15 years of age.

15. **Black men and women** were 64 percent less likely to report painful heart attack symptoms than whites, and 50 percent more likely to attribute their discomfort to non-cardiac causes. *(American Journal of Public Health)*

16. Coronary artery disease and cancer incidence is skyrocketing in certain countries in Asia and the Middle East.

17. Coronary artery bypass **treats only a few inches** of the arteries whereas atherosclerosis can affect 65 miles of arteries.

18. Dr. Dean Ornish's Lifestyle Heart Trial, which used a ten percent-fat vegetarian diet with exercise and stress management **showed regression** in coronary heart disease in one year with increased regression in four years, compared to a control group following an American Heart Association Step-2 Diet.

19. In the Framingham Study, women who were obese were twice as likely to develop coronary heart disease as those who were not.

20. Dr. Antonio Gotto's study with Lovastatin shows the drug prevents heart attacks, sudden deaths and angina in healthy people whose **cholesterol levels are nearly normal.**

21. A recent American Medical Association News article described a number of newly developed cholesterol-lowering drugs which in clinical trials **reduced** the incidence of **stroke** by 29%, **reduced cardiovascular disease** by 28%, and **reduced mortality** risk by 22%.

22. West of Scotland study, prevention of a first heart attack with **Pravastatin,** (Pravachol®) **heart attacks down by 31%.**

23. 4 S study using **Simvastatin** (Zocor®) showed **decrease** in heart disease **deaths by 42%**, over all deaths by 30% and bypass and angioplasty by 37%.

24. Fluvastatin slows the progression of coronary artery disease in patients with mild to moderate hypercholesterolemia.

25. Evidence for more benefits of cholesterol lowering drugs. (*Journal of the American Medical Association – J.A.M.A. – Oct. 1, 1997.*)

26. Diabetes produces a **five-fold increase** in cardiovascular risk **in women,** compared to a two-fold increase in men. (*Johns Hopkins Health After 50 Medical Letter*)

27. In a 1995 study conducted in Lyon, France, men and women who had suffered heart attacks and were assigned to follow a Mediterranean Diet reduced the risk of another heart attack by 70 percent. (New evidence -Mediterranean diet decreases incidence of cancer.)

28. Polyunsaturated fatty acids are more prone to oxidation. Excess polyunsaturates can accelerate aging.

29. Pima Indians are known to have an extremely high diabetes rate among their population, but a lower rate of heart disease compared to that of Americans.

30. Asian Indians, who are non-smokers, do not consume alcohol, and are vegetarians, have an extremely high incidence of heart disease.

31. People who ate more fish in Finland had higher heart disease because of mercury contamination.

32. People who ate more fish in Tanzania had a higher concentration of N-3 polyunsaturated fatty acids, lower blood pressure and lower plasma lipid concentration.

33. Japanese women who eat fatty fish had lower incidence of breast cancer.

34. Fish oil decreases triglyceride level.

35. Fish consumption decreased the incidence of sudden cardiac death.

36. Increased fish consumption **decreased** cardiac death and **all-cause mortality**. (*J.A.M.A., Jan. 7, 1998*)

37. Moderate alcohol intake decreases coronary artery disease.

38. A study of **wine drinkers** in the city of Copenhagen, Denmark revealed **lower overall mortality** compared with people who consumed other beverages.

39. A new study on relative efficacy of water, beer, pure alcohol, whiskey, white wine and red wine in the prevention of coronary artery disease showed **red wine to be the best; water and beer had no effect on prevention.**

40. Beer bingeing increases fatal heart attacks. Dose-responsive increase was observed between beer quantity and all cause mortality **with three bottles of beer per session**. (*British Medical Journal, Oct. 4, 1997*)

41. Three cups of red/purple grape juice has same benefit as one cup of red wine without the side effects of alcohol.

42. A one-percent drop in adult smoking would result in 98,100 fewer hospitalizations for heart attacks and strokes; 13,100 fewer deaths attributed to heart attacks and strokes and 3.2 billion dollars in avoided medical costs over a seven year period. (*J.A.M.A., Jan. 14, 1998*)

43. Smoking causes premature accelerated, irreversible hardening of the coronary arteries. (*J.A.M.A., Jan. 14, 1998*)

44. Smoking accelerates new coronary lesion progression.

45. Active smokers' arteries hardened 50% faster than those of non-smokers, and ex-smokers' arteries hardened 25% faster than those of non-smokers. (*J.A.M.A., Jan. 14, 1998*)

46. Cigarette smoking is blamed for 55% of the coronary events in adults younger than the age of 55.

47. Lovastatin attenuates the progression of coronary atherosclerosis and delays or prevents the development of new lesions in smokers. (*Cardiology 1997*).

48. Passive smoke lowers HDL (good cholesterol) level in children, thereby increases risk.

49. Passive smoking in the workplace increases risk of heart disease.

50. Cigarette smoking increases fibrinogen levels which increases blood clot formation.

51. Homocysteine causes heart disease — several studies.

52. High homocysteine level increases the risk of heart attacks in women.

53. Increased Homocysteine is found in post-menopausal women.

54. Homocysteine and carotid artery disease lead to strokes.

55. Homocysteine and deep vein thrombosis causing clots in the leg veins predispos-

19

ing to pulmonary embolism. (*New England Journal of Medicine*)

56. Severe lower limb atherosclerotic disease in young patients with high homocysteine levels.

57. Elevated homocysteine causes systolic hypertension. (*Physicians Weekly 4/29/96*)

58. While men are sensitive to high LDL cholesterol, women are more sensitive to **low HDL**, and **borderline high triglyceride**. (*Johns Hopkins Health After 50 Medical Letter, June, 1998*)

59. In a study of 2906 middle-aged and older men followed for eight years even levels of **142-200 mg/dl of triglyceride** was a **strong predictor independent** of any other risk factors **including HDL**. (*Published in Circulation – Reported in Physicians' Weekly, May 11, 1998.*)

60. Case control trials of vitamin E have consistently demonstrated a lower coronary risk for both men and women with the highest vitamin E intake. (*Ray W. Squires, Ph.D.*) Caution! Excessive vitamin E intake may cause bleeding! (*Dr. Pai*)

61. A Finnish study of 29,000 men ages 50-69 who took 50 I.U. of vitamin E each day for five to eight years had 32 percent fewer diagnoses of prostate cancer and 41 percent fewer prostate cancer deaths, compared to men who had no vitamin E.

62. Left Atrial enlargement is an independent risk factor for strokes.

63. Syndrome X - Atherogenic Dyslipidemia. Fasting hyperinsulinemia, higher fasting concentration of triglycerides, and cholesterol with lower HDL, 75% had abnormal cardiac adrenergic tone, 76% had cerebral perfusion abnormalities.

64. Lipoprotein E (especially E4) are associated with increased cardiovascular risk.

65. Lipoprotein B (APO B) predictor of heart disease risk.

66. Lipoprotein A [LP(a)] independent risk factor of heart disease. [LP(a)] is **atherogenic and thrombogenic.**

67. Small, dense triglyceride-rich particles – pattern B-associated with low HDL, high insulin level and increased fat in blood after a meal, present in 50% of the men with heart disease. Increased risk is threefold.

68. Vitamin C and E diminish arterial constriction response after a fatty meal. (Also decreases skin cancer after exposure to sun)

69. Low fat, and fat free food snack explosion has increased the consumption of carbohydrates which increase triglycerides. (Similar to rice induced triglyceride increase in the East).

70. A decreased concentration of HDL can predispose people to stroke even when their LDL cholesterol is acceptably low. (*Minneapolis V.A.M.C. study – Tufts Univ. HN Letter December 1997*).

71. High cholesterol levels change vascular response to exercise even in normal arteries.

72. Patients with periodontal disease have increased incidence of coronary artery disease. (Dental plaque may lead to coronary plaques!)

73. Chlamydia infection causing coronary atherosclerosis shown by Muhlestein and

74. Treatment of **high-coronary-risk** patient with severe coronary artery disease with **azithromycin dramatically decreased the risk.** *British study by Dr. Sandeep Gupta.*

75. **High-risk cardiac patients** treated with **roxithromycin** and **standard antithrombotic** therapy had **reduced adverse cardiac events.** *Dr. Enrique Gurfinkel.*

76. CMV infection causes early closure of coronary arteries after balloon angioplasty.

77. A laser may be used to drill holes in the heart muscle when very bad coronary artery disease is not bypassable. Thus, the heart muscle gets blood directly from the heart cavity. *(Harvard Heart Letter, March, 1998)*

78. Mental stress causes myocardial ischemia. *(J.A.M.A., June 5, 1996)*

79. Mental stress can cause an exaggerated systolic blood pressure response in hypercholesterolemic patients.

80. Anger – **a dose-responsive** relation between the **level of anger** and overall coro-

colleagues from Salt Lake City, Utah (*Cardiology 1997*).

nary artery disease risk shown by Kawachi and colleagues in Boston, Massachusetts. (*Cardiology-1997*)

81. Emotionally defensive people (people who deny the presence of socially undesirable characteristics in one self) may be exposed to greater surges in blood pressure **and a greater risk of heart attack.**

82. Depression is associated with increased incidence of heart disease.

83. The S.S.R.I. antidepressant Paroxetine acid (Paxil) is safer than the tricyclic antidepressant Nortriptyline, which can increase heart rate in patients with ischemic heart disease. However, Paroxetine is not risk-free, as it can interact with other heart medications.

84. Self-centered people with heart disease who are preoccupied with "I-Me-Myself" have more cardiac events. (*Study by Larry Sherwitz at U.C.S.F.*)

85. Veterans with post-traumatic stress disorder have a 62% increase in cardiovascular disease.

86. A temporary increase in incidence of heart attacks during major earthquakes.

87. Mustard oil contains 7% erusic acid. **More than 2% erusic acid** can **cause cardiac conduction defects**, some of which require a pacemaker.

88. Fifty percent of all pacemakers implanted in India are in the state of West Bengal (Mother Teresa's home state) where mustard oil is the most common cooking medium.

89. A parasite can cause heart block (*Chagas Disease*) for which patients need a pacemaker.

90. Cellular telephones have been found to cause interference with pacemaker function. This is especially **true of digital cell phones** when they are operated **near the pacemaker!** *COMMENT: Be careful you don't "reach out and hurt someone!"* –Dr. Pai

91. Prolonged conversation with lateral flexion of the neck on a cordless phone causing carotid artery dissection (major cause of stroke in young people) in a young woman. (*New England Journal of Medicine, Feb. 13, 1997*).

92. Ephedrine from ephedra used as a metabolic stimulant can raise blood pressure and risk of heart attack and stroke. (Present in some herbal weight loss products.)

93. Cocaine causes high blood pressure, irregular heartbeat, stroke, and sudden cardiac death.

94. Prolonged and heavy use of nasal vaso-constrictor drops can cause severe hypertension, stroke, heart attack and death.

95. Elevated C-reactive protein is associated with coronary artery disease. (in men and women)

96. Men with the **highest C-reactive protein levels** were found to be **three times more likely** to have heart attack than men with the lowest levels. (*Harvard Mens' Health Watch, Feb., 1998*) (*Also increases mortality in unstable angina.*)

97. High levels of fibrinogen are associated with the winter season, high body weight, diabetes, cigarette smoking, hyperlipidemia, menopause, and inflammation or infection.

98. Low levels of fibrinogen have been observed with the summer season, regular exercise, hormone replacement therapy, high HDL cholesterol, moderate alcohol consumption, and a diet rich in polyunsaturated fatty acids.

99. Moderate exercise decreases fibrinogen. Vigorous exercise raises it.

100. In a 12-year study of 700 retired men in their 60's, 70's and 80's, those who jogged two miles each day cut their risk of dying in half, compared with those who walked less than one mile. The more the men walked, the greater the benefit. (*Tufts University Health Letter, March, 1998.*)

101. Strenuous exercise provokes rupture of vulnerable plaques in dyslipidimec men with severe coronary disease. (*American Heart Association Abstract #469, November 10, 1997 - Virmani, Malcom et al*)

102. Harvard researchers studying 46,000 men of ages 40 to 75 for eight years found that those who exercised the most had the least risk for gallstones.

103. A recent study published in the European Heart Journal found that **family history** may be a **more significant risk factor for for women** than **for men.**

104. **Diabetes and obesity** are more prevalent among the **African Americans**, especially **women**.

105. Abnormal clotting factors and high P.A.I. levels increase the incidence of heart disease.

106. A recent University of Alabama study of 327,000 men and women of all ages treated at about 1,500 U.S. hospitals from 1994 to 1996 **revealed that women are almost 50 percent more likely than men to die from heart attacks.** The reason for this, in part, is owing to the fact that the average woman who suffers her first heart attack is typically 10 years older than the average man who has his first episode. Such women also are more likely to have other complicating diseases, like diabetes and high blood pressure. The smaller size of women's coronary arteries compared to men's also makes them more difficult to treat.

107. **Women typically take an hour longer to get to the hospital following a heart attack** and are **treated less urgently** by emergency room personnel once they arrive, according to a report presented at a meeting of the American College of Cardiology in

Atlanta on April 1, 1998. One reason for this, according to Dr. Sandra Gan of the Swedish Medical Center in Seattle, is that women are less likely to suffer the crushing chest pain that is a hallmark of most heart attacks in men. Instead, they may have more **ambiguous symptoms**, such as shortness of breath, **pain in the neck or jaw, or symptoms that resemble gas pains.**

108. Heart diseases in women can be more accurately diagnosed using the QT dispersion on the electrocardiogram. (*Dr. R. Pai, Loma Linda University School of Medicine, California*)

109. Emergency room rapid testing for troponin T or I for early detection of myocardial cell injury in acute coronary syndromes. (*New England Journal of Medicine, December 4, 1997*)

110. Patients who were on Fen-Phen need to have their echocardiogram done to rule out possible heart valve damage.

111. If patients have heart valve damage they need to take prophylactic antibiotics before dental procedures or certain operations.

112. Fen-Phen causes heart valve damage and pulmonary hypertension; also, animal studies with Fenfluramine have shown brain damage. The heart valve damage resembles changes which occur in carcinoid syndrome or ergot-induced heart valve damage.

113. Infants with low birth weight have a higher incidence of coronary artery disease.

114. Cold weather increases mortality from ischemic heart disease, cerebrovascular disease, respiratory disease when people do not use appropriate warm clothing.

115. Intravascular **coronary radiotherapy** treatments have demonstrated a significant reduction in proliferation after balloon angioplasty and stenting thus **reduce the incidence of restenosis.**

116. Probucol, a powerful antioxidant, prevents restenosis after balloon angioplasty, but only if therapy is started four weeks prior to the procedure. **1.** Works better than antioxidant vitamins!—Impractical, because most angioplasties are emergency procedures. **2. Other antioxidants diminish Probucol effects.**

117. Hardened fat, hardened arteries: – Trans fats have **adverse effects** on cholesterol profiles. (*New England Journal of Medicine, November 20, 1997*)

118. Trans-fats appear to raise lipoprotein LP(a) levels and may increase thrombogenesis. (*Donald Hensrud, M.D., Mayo Clinic Teleconference.*)

119. Hardened Heart Valves have bone tissue components. A University of Pennsylvania study headed by Dr. Emile Mohler, III, found ossification in 30 of the 220 aortic and mitral valves. There was cartilaginous tissue in four valves, osteoclasts in 11, and mineralized tissue in 95 percent of the specimens. Only 22 percent had rheumatic fever, 46 percent had coronary disease; 11 percent had narrowed carotid arteries; and 9 percent had peripheral vascular disease; 48 percent had hypertension; 51 percent smoking; 23 percent hypercholesterolemia; and 17 percent had diabetes. Last year the same group found osteopontin in calcified valves, suggesting **valvular ossification is an active process** and not a degenerative process, pointing towards possible new preventive or protective therapies. (*Physicians' Weekly, May 11, 1998.*)

120. Researchers from Tokyo's Kasai Gakuin University found eating animal protein led to a greater loss of calcium than eating plant protein. The more protein the volunteers ate, the greater was their loss of calcium. (*American Journal of Clinical Nutrition, March, 1998.*)

121. Replacing saturated and trans unsaturated fats with unhydrogenated monounsaturated and polyunsaturated fats are more effective in preventing coronary artery disease in women than reducing overall fat intake. (*New England Journal of Medicine, Nov. 20, 1997.*)

122. Several studies have shown that when blacks and whites have the same access to medical care both groups have comparable survival rates and a similar response to treatment.

123. A high-fat meal induces changes in blood rheology (flow) in patients with obstructive coronary artery disease and may contribute to worsening anginal symptoms at rest. (*Dr. R. Baliga, London. Supplement to Circulation, Oct. 20,1997*)

COMMENT: *Viscous blood means 1. Sluggish flow and 2. In a new study speeds up hardening of the arteries.*

124. MAO (monoaminooxidase) inhibitors can cause fatal interactions with tyramine found in common foods like cheddar cheese, many other cheeses, avocado, pepperoni, salami, soy sauce, canned and overripe figs, chicken liver, Chianti, Drambuie® liqueur, large quantities of chocolate or caffeine, broad bean pods (fava beans), yeast concentrates, other drugs like demerol, dextromethorphan (cough syrup), cocaine and ephedrine. The antibiotic furazolidine, and the anticancer drug procarbazine may also act like MAO inhibitors. (*People's Guide to Drug Interactions – Teresa and Joe Graedon Ph.D.*)

125. A study of Japanese who regularly supplement their diets with **green tea antioxidants** (Epigallocatechin-3-Gallate and epicathecin-3-Gallate) were shown to **have lower overall cancer rate** even though they **admittedly smoked twice as many ciga-**

rettes every day as their American counterparts. *(Tufts University Health & Nutrition Letter - August 1997)*

126. Japanese men who drink green tea also have **lower LDL cholesterol** and **triglyceride levels**, and **higher HDL levels**, and consequently, a lower overall rate of heart disease. *(Cardiology, 1996)*

127. Ten cups of green tea decreased liver enzymes aspartate aminotransferase, alanine transferase and ferritin. *(Cardiology, 1996)*

128. Increased iron intake causes increased heart disease. This cause has been debated for several years, but has been reconfirmed using new, accurate methods of iron assay. *(Physicians' Weekly, Jan. 19, 1998)*

129. Iron overload and release from tissue stores accelerate lipid peroxidation.

COMMENT: Contrary to public opinion, increased iron intake will not make you a "magnetic personality... but you may rust in peace! (Rusting is the layman's term for oxidation.) Iron overload increases 1. Cancer. (NHANES III) and 2. Heart Disease (many studies.) 3. N.I.D. Diabetes Mellitus. (BMJ)

130. Among smokers who consume ten cups of green tea, the lipid peroxidase enzyme

34

was reduced to the level of non-smokers.

131. Iron Overload Disease (Hereditary hemochromatosis) is more common than many doctors think it is, and **goes undiagnosed.** The Center for Disease Control and Prevention estimates **one in 200 Americans have hemochromatosis, making it the most common inherited disorder – 50 times more common than previously thought.** (*Another good reason to donate blood often and stay off iron supplements! – Dr. Pai*)

132. F2 Isoprostane formation (derived from arachidonic acid) is believed to be a marker for human vascular disease. Levels of this substance can be measured in the urine, providing a non-invasive index of lipid peroxidations in the setting of cardiac reperfusion injury, with or without cardiovascular risk factors including cigarette smoking, diabetes mellitus, and hypercholesterolemia. (*Patrono, C. & G. Fitzgerald, Journal of Arteriosclerosis, Thrombosis & Vascular Biology, 17:11.*)

133. Though black men have twice the incidence of hypertension compared to white men, the prevalence of coronary artery disease is two to three times greater in White men compared to Black men. (*A 1960 study cited in Cardiology, 1996*)

134. It has been observed that the **French consume more saturated fat** than Americans do, but **have less heart disease.**

135. When the Communist regime ended recently in Soviet Russia and countries of the former U.S.S.R., the incidence of heart disease skyrocketed due to the change in lifestyles. (*Remember: the genetics and other risk factors remained the same!*)

136. Coronary plaques were virtually absent in people who had undergone starvation during World War II. However, they made a quick comeback during the years of postwar prosperity.

137. The incidence of heart disease was much higher in British bus drivers compared to conductors in a double-decker bus, even though their race and dietary habits were similar. (The conductors had more exercise; the drivers had more stress.)

138. Liquid protein diet and starvation can increase the QT interval on the EKG, which can lead to a fatal arrythmia called Torsades de pointes (a type of ventricular tachycardia).

139. Torsades de pointes can also be caused when antihistamines such as terfenedine (Seldane®) or astemizole (Hismanal®) are used with erythromycin, resulting in sudden death. Torsades de pointes is also caused by Propulsid® (Cisapride), with certain antibiotics and antifungals.

140. Researchers in Boston found that the **risk** of a heart attack was **16 times** greater for patients with the highest triglyceride-to-HDL ratio when compared to those with the lowest TGL:HDL ratios. (*Circulation, Oct. 21, 1997*)

141. Heart-failure patients on a low-dose ACE inhibitor (lisinopril) had an 8:1 higher risk of death compared to patients who were given high dosages of this common anti-hypertensive drug. (*Dr. Milton Packer, reporting at American College of Cardiology Meeting in Atlanta, April 1, 1998*)

142. Patients with non insulin dependent diabetes and hypertension on calcium-channel blockers had more fatal and non-fatal heart attacks compared to patients on ACE inhibitors. (*New Eng J of Med, March 5, 1998*)

143. Baseline-soluble intercellular adhesion molecule-1 (SICAM-1) levels that exceed the 75th percentile were highly correlated with the risk of myocardial infarction. (*LANCET, Jan. 10, 1998*)

144. Microalbuminuria predicts the presence and severity of coronary artery disease. (*Reported by Dr. Katherine Tuttle, Heart Institute of Spokane, WA, at the April 1, 1998 meeting of the American College of Cardiologists, Atlanta, GA*)

145. Quebec Cardiovascular Study showed that standard risk factors of high triglycerides and LDL and low HDL had a **4.4-fold** risk compared to men with none of the risk factors. However, the risk was **20- fold** for men with a triad of elevated fasting insulin, Apolipoprotein B and small, dense LDL particles. In addition to the triad, if patient had impaired glucose tolerance, greater postprandial lipemia and high concentrations of fibrinogen and plasminogen activator inhibitor Type 1, the **risk hits heights that merit aggressive intervention**. (*Physicians' Weekly, Feb. 2, 1998*)

146. Physical characteristics which have increased heart disease incidence include Truncal Obesity, Male Pattern Baldness, Ear Lobe Crease, Snoring and Sleep Apnea.

147. Most Americans do not get enough sleep, which could be a contributing factor to heart disease.

148. During National Sleep Awareness Week in March, 1998, the National Sleep Foundation released data that suggest average Americans run up a "sleep debt" of about 500 hours a year. Contrary to popular belief, adults do not require less sleep as they get older.

149. Snoring and sleep apnea are symptoms of problems that require medical attention, and many people simply ignore them.

150. Important Facts: The human body never fully adjusts to night shift work, and sleep disorders do not go away without treatment. The human body cannot function properly with one or two fewer hours of sleep a night than it needs.

151. Lack of sleep is linked to weight gain, depression, lethargy, memory loss, risk of infection (due to lowered immunity) and aging - not to mention the **100,000 car crashes due to sleepy drivers.**

152. 70% of the **air crashes** are due to human error, some due to sleep deprivation among **airline pilots. Sleep deprivation** has also been blamed for inappropriate care by **resident doctors.**

153. Sleepiness, driving and motor vehicle crashes *James M. Lyznicki MS MPH J.A.M.A., June 17, 1998; 1908-1913* Driver sleepiness is a causative factor in **1% to 3% of all US motor vehicle crashes.**

COMMENT: If you are sleepy lowering windows or turning up the radio does not help - Get off the road and sleep in a safe place. Never use cruise control when sleepy. -Dr. Pai

154. Exercise caution while exercising - many people who undertake sudden vigorous exercise can have many sports related injuries besides risking plaque rupture.

155. Prolonged bending forward and bike riding can cause impotence because of decreased blood flow to the penis.

COMMENT: (Vicious cycle indeed!) Back to the easy rider bikes... Lean back and relax.

156. HARDENED ARTERIES–BRITTLE BONES? Lipid oxidation products have opposite effects on calcifying vascular cell and bone cell differentiation. ...A possible explanation for the PARADOX OF ARTERIAL CALCIFICATION IN OSTEOPOROTIC PATIENTS. (*Source: Parhami et al, UCLA Study, Journal of Arteriosclerosis, Thrombosis and Vascular Biology, 17:4, April, 1997*)

Remember, **many people who appeared to be in excellent physical shape**, like **Arthur Ashe** and **Sergei Grinkov**, had **heart disease**. Never say, "This can never happen to me." (*Remember the Titanic*) The most significant causes of heart disease are lack of exercise, lifestyle and diet.

Why talk about sleep deprivation and accidents in a book on prevention of heart disease? Because cardiac contusion (a bruised heart) is preventable! so is injury to other vital organs.

The following treatment plan is not meant for pregnant women or women who can become pregnant. *Please consult your physician.*

FACTORS KNOWN TO PREVENT CORONARY ARTERY DISEASE... SOME ALONE OR IN COMBINATION:

A. Low-fat vegetarian diet

A1. Increase intake of pesticide free and preservative free fruits and vegetables.

B. Fiber (Increased fiber intake)

C. Vitamin C at least 500mg (natural preferred)

D1. Control of Diabetes

D2. Drugs/Dietary Supplements: Aspirin, ACE inhibitors, L-Arginine, Beta-blockers, B-6 and B-12 vitamins, Coenzyme Q-10 (*Cardiology, 1997*), cholesterol-lowering statins and intermittent therapy with antibiotics. (Don't mix certain statins with **certain antibiotics.** Stop one temporarily before taking the other.) Azithromycin or roxithromycin for chlamydia. Patients on Hismanal®, Propulsid®, Mevacor® or Zocor® **SHOULD NOT TAKE** erythromycin, ketoconozale, or related drugs because of dangerous drug interactions. Check with your pharmacist about all possible drug interactions between **drugs and drugs, drugs and foods, and drugs, foods, vitamins, herbals and disease processes.**

Grapefruit juice can increase levels of Lovastatin (Mevacor®) when patient is on high dose Lovastatin. Low doses of Mevacor® and Zocor® aren't likely to cause problems. (*Prescribers' Newsltr July 1998*)

Also note the safe doses for vitamins. For example, more than 100 mg per day of vitamin B6 can induce sensory neuropathy.

E1. Vitamin E (at least 400 I.U. daily)
(mixed tocopherol preferred)

E2. Exercise

F1. Folic acid (at least 400 mcg to 1000 mcg daily) – along with B12 supplements (NOTE: More than 1000 mcg of folic acid can mask vitamin B12 deficiency, which can lead to tingling, numbness, irreversible neurological damage; Subacute combined degeneration of the spinal cord – even with a normal blood picture.)

F2. Fish (increased consumption of non-polluted fish)

F3. Fat (monounsaturated to substitute for saturated fats)

F4. Flavinoids - increased intake.

G1. Gene therapy to bypass coronary blockages. (This has shown promising results recently in leg arteries!)

G2. Gene therapy to prevent intimal hyperplasia.

G3. Glycoprotein IIb/IIIa blockade in prevention of complications of coronary interventional procedures and in the treatment of acute coronary syndromes.

H1. Control of Hypertension

H2. Hormone replacement therapy (in women) (New controversy see page 91)

L. Lycopene - Protects against heart disease and prostate cancer

M1. Mediterranean diet (Mediterranean "Peasant" Diet)

M2. Milano mutant gene

O. Omega-3 fatty acids

P. Decrease pollution risk

Q. Quit smoking!

S1. Statins: CHOLESTEROL-LOWERING STATINS REDUCE LDL CHOLESTEROL. STATINS STABILIZE THE PLAQUE. If no contraindications, statin therapy, even in people with "normal" **cholesterol. (Remember: Yesterday's "normal" cholesterol 250 mg/dl – is today's high cholesterol.) 200mg/dl** (with no other cardiac risk factors) is the presently accepted total cholesterol level (which may have a downward revision soon.) Even though a Triglyceride level of 200mg/dl or less is considered normal (*National Cholesterol Education Programs A.T.P.II 93*) Many authorities think that a lower triglyceride level is desirable.

S2.

Stress reduction therapy

Most common cause of heart attack: Plaque Rupture.

Goals of therapy: 1. Plaque Stabilization. 2. Restore endothelial function.

Most effective class of drugs for **prevention: Statins.** Some of the risk factors for coronary artery disease pose the same risks for cancer. The goal of my program is not only to prevent heart disease but also reverse it. The biggest problem with coronary artery disease and cancer is the attitude, "It can never happen to me".

S3. Participation in social, and or religious and or community support groups.

S4. Sitostanol - Pine margarine

S5. Increase soy protein intake

LDL Cholesterol = Total Cholesterol - HDL - (Triglycerides ÷ 5)

If Total Cholesterol = 200mg/dL
and *("Good" Cholesterol)* HDL = 40mg/dL
and Triglycerides = 150mg/dL

then, LDL Cholesterol = 200 - 40 - (150/5)
("Bad" Cholesterol)   or, 200 - 40 - (30)
or, 160 - 30 = 130 mg/dL

NOTE: This formula applies only if the triglyceride level is below 400mg/dL.

National Cholesterol Education Program
Recommendations for Lipid Therapy
ATPII 1993 Based on LDL Cholesterol

DRUG TREATMENT

	Initiating Level	Minimal Goal
Without CHD or two other risk factors	> 190mg/dL	< 160mg/dL
Without CHD two other risk factors	> 160mg/dL	< 130mg/dL
With CHD	> 130mg/dL	<100mg/dL

The narrowing of the arteries takes place over a long period of time, and, just like highways which, when closed, lead to the development of alternate routes, so do the coronary arteries. These alternate routes are called collaterals.

In patients who experience plaque rupture, **a heart attack occurs without warning – even in a "healthy" patient whose recent EKG, Echocardiogram and Stress Tests may have been normal.** Even the ultra-fast CT scan which can pick all calcified plaques non-invasively would not show a non-calcified plaque.

A majority of heart attacks occur because of a phenomenon known as "plaque rupture." The fatty plaque in the coronary artery resembles an acne lesion with a very thin cap or a snow-capped peak. The rupture of this cap causes clot-forming fatty material to be deposited in the artery. The formation of the clot seals off the artery (old term: coronary thrombosis), causing a heart attack. **Somehow, the unstable plaques are**

seen in wider arteries (50 percent narrowing versus 70 percent). In the wider arteries the plaques are subjected to a larger shearing force of the circulating blood. **Plaque rupture can also occur by a process called apoptosis** (programmed cell death). **Prior to a heart attack such patients are symptom-free,** whereas patients with 70 percent or greater narrowing have anginal symptoms (i.e., chest pain and shortness of breath).

In plaque erosion, the "snow cap" is lost, and when a plaque ruptures a volcano-like eruption causes the fatty clot-promoting matter to be extruded into the artery, thus clotting-off of the artery and causing heart attacks. In plaque erosion the clot is on the surface of the plaque, whereas in plaque rupture the clot is formed in the fatty core of the plaque. (Analogy: In plaque erosion the clot is from the top of the mountain peak, whereas in plaque rupture the clot is from deep inside the mountain.)

The plaque may have a thick, fibrous structure analogous to a steel helmet, which may prevent plaque rupture, or, conversely, it might have a thin cap analogous to a shower cap, which is quite prone to rupture.

Plaque stabilization is the goal of lipid-lowering therapy, usually with statin drugs. Supplementing certain antioxidants should aid this process. (example Vit E, green tea)

Decreasing high homocysteine levels is another priority, as homocysteine makes the inner lining of the arteries "sticky" and more prone to plaque and clot formation. The treatment is inexpensive and includes folic acid and certain other vitamins B-6 and B-12.

Aspirin decreases inflammation and platelet "stickiness," hence it has been recommended as an aid in the prevention of heart attacks.

FACTORS INCREASING STRESS

➡ thin fibrous cap
large lipid pool
less stenotic lesions
➡ (ester/free) cholesterol

FACTORS WEAKENING THE CAP

⬅ collagen synthesis
➡ collagen degradation
➡ macrophages, T-cells
⬅ smooth muscle cells

Source: Lee, Richard T. and Peter Libby, The Unstable Atheroma. The Journal of Arteriosclerosis, Thrombosis and Vascular Biology, 17:10, October, 1997.

HOMOCYSTEINE: A CAUSE OF ATHERO-SCLEROSIS (HARDENING OF THE ARTERIES)

In the mid-1960's Dr. Kilmer McCully was intrigued by two children who died as a result of Homocysteinuria, a condition in which high levels of homocysteine exist in the blood and urine. In both cases the direct cause of death was severe atherosclerosis, or hardening of the arteries —a condition usually seen only in patients of advanced age.

In animal studies the toxic effect of homocysteine was detoxified primarily by folic acid and also vitamins B-6 and B- 12.

In the human body homocysteine is produced from methionine, which is a constituent of the protein (not fat or carbohydrate) component of meat, milk, cheese and eggs. The damage caused by homocysteine to the arterial inner wall resulting in atherosclerosis has **been called "protein intoxication" by Dr. McCully.**

The homocysteine damage to the artery can be compared to a dent on the body of an automobile resulting from an accident. Oxidized cholesterol builds up in this "dent" much like the buildup of rust in the dent of a car door or fender. The common-sense, take-home message here is: If you can prevent a dent in the artery by taking folic acid and vitamins B-6 and B-12, you can thus minimize damage to your arteries from cholesterol buildup. New studies show folic acid and vitamin B-6 protect the artery from homocysteine damage. However, folic acid given alone may mask vitamin B-12 deficiency. That is why vitamin B-12 is given in combination with folic acid and vitamin B-6. Before starting folic acid therapy, check a serum B-12 level, as folic acid can mask the serious neurological manifestation of B-12 deficiency called subacute combined degeneration of the spinal cord. **[The neurological damage can happen even with a normal hematological picture** *(New England Journal of Medicine, April 2, 1998).]*

University of Minnesota scientists think that homocysteine might be a result rather than a cause of heart disease; but they did notice that people with the highest B-6 blood levels had one third the risk of people with the lowest B-6 levels.

*NOTE: Homocysteine makes arteries "sticky," thus promoting cholesterol buildup. **Homocysteine could increase the risk of clotting, both in the arteries and veins.***

53

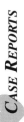

Case Reports

Case Report #1 A 47-year-old male patient with severe 3-vessel coronary artery disease suffered a heart attack affecting a small area of the heart muscle. The patient was a heavy smoker, and was considered to be a candidate for an emergency coronary artery bypass graft. The patient's surgery was put off for personal reasons. He was treated medically, discharged and asked to return for bypass surgery at a later date.

The patient quit smoking and started taking a statin drug to lower cholesterol. He returned after 6 months for his bypass surgery. A heart catheterization revealed that all three arteries had opened up and he did not need coronary artery bypass surgery. The patient and his doctors were amazed. The patient was discharged and he continued to take the cholesterol lowering statin drug.

Case Report #2 A 45-year-old obese patient with coronary artery disease had a balloon angioplasty to open a blocked coronary artery. The balloon only temporarily opened the coronary artery, which closed in a matter of months.

The patient had a second balloon angioplasty to open the same coronary artery, after which he was put on cholesterol-lowering drugs. Unknown to his doctors, the patient started taking vitamin E, about which he learned from his friends. After this the patient had a fall and he **gained 50 pounds** as he could not exercise **because of the leg injury.**

Eight months later the patient had an episode of chest discomfort for which he had repeat heart catheterization. His doctors were surprised to discover that **his blocked artery had opened** up in spite of a **50-pound weight gain.** The cause of his chest pain this time was found to be non-cardiac in origin. Subsequently, the patient had two more heart catheterizations (by different cardiologists) for chest discomfort, and there was no evidence of blockages.

RECENT ADVANCES IN THE UNDER-STANDING OF THE MECHANISMS OF THE CAUSES OF HEART ATTACK:

For the last several decades, doctors have been taught that heart attacks occur mostly in the severely-narrowed (70 percent or above) coronary arteries. However, recent evidence suggests the contrary. An example of this is the following case.

CASE REPORT #3 A patient with known two-vessel coronary artery disease was brought to the emergency room following a heart attack. His third coronary artery prior to the emergency room visit had been diagnosed as "normal." The muscular walls of his heart supplied by the severely-narrowed arteries were contracting sluggishly. The muscular wall of the heart that was supplied by the "normal" artery was beating normally prior to the heart attack. After tests were conducted, much to the physicians' surprise, **the heart attack affected the "normal" artery and the muscle wall** (the only portion of the heart that was beating normally prior to the heart attack) was not moving at all. The other sluggishly-contracting walls were still contracting sluggishly. The total effect was poor pump function with inadequate perfusion to the various organs of the body.

COMMENT: Don't cheat on your diet and exercise programs, as weight gain can reduce the efficacy of statin drugs. Weight gain also increased the risk for other diseases. -Dr. Pai

157. During a trial run of a HDTV broadcast in Texas many pacemakers were reprogrammed, causing temporary malfunction. (CNN) *(Pacemaker malfunction is also caused by anti-theft devices used in stores.) (NOTE: the technology of tomorrow may interfere with the medical devices of today. Such broadcasts of HDTV should be halted until a clearer picture emerges about possible pacemaker malfunction).*

158. According to a study published in the *Journal of the National Cancer Institute* **(Dec 17, 1997) green tea** has been shown to protect **against all stages of cancer including the start, growth and spread of cancer.**

159. In various articles, USA Today reports that the use of Vitamin E supplements reduces **the risk of prostate cancer, heart disease and Alzheimer's Disease.**

160. Four million new cases of sexually transmitted chlamydia occurred last year *(headline news).* (***Remember***: *chlamydia can cause heart disease!)*

161. More studies are needed to determine if non-sexual chlamydial diseases (*which are very common in some countries*) cause heart disease.

162. In the 1960's, due to the widespread use of erythromycin and tetracycline as the major antibiotics for most infections, there was a significant decrease in coronary artery disease. This was further decreased when salyicilates were added during food processing. (Erythromycin and tetracycline kill the chlamydia microorganisms, and salyicilates work like aspirin.)

163. Pravachol® (pravastatin) and Zocor® (simvastatin) recently were approved for use in the **prevention of stroke.** These statins lower **the risk of stroke** by almost A THIRD in patients with heart disease – even in some heart patients with AVERAGE **cholesterol.** (*Prescribers Nwsltr, May, 98*)

164. Several drugs, foods and food supplements can interact with each other, sometimes causing fatal consequences.

Posicor® (Mibefradil) (Blood Pressure and antiangina drug) withdrawn because of serious side effects due to drug interactions even days after it was stopped.

165. The drugs of tomorrow may interact with the drugs of today, possibly with unusual side-effects which may be fatal. Newspaper and magazine reports in the last decade have documented numerous tragic occurrences of vehicle drivers, heavy equipment operators, and even airline pilots who have died on the job as a result of adverse drug interactions.

COMMENT: Several years ago, for example, the pilot of a commercial aircraft who was taking oral hypoglycemic medication (without medical supervision) attended a party and had a few drinks the night before a scheduled flight. The next morning while he was piloting the aircraft he had an antabuse type of reaction resulting in hallucinations, and, despite warnings from his co-pilot, crashed the airliner, which caused the loss of more than 200 lives.

166. 106,000 deaths in 1994 were discovered to have resulted from adverse drug reaction (ADR), making ADR one of the leading causes of death, after heart disease, cancer and stroke. These are neither prescribing, dispensing or non-compliance errors (taking more or less of a drug than the prescribed amount), or therapeutic failures or intentional and accidental poisoning (overdose) and drug abuse, but rather noxious, unintended and undesired effect of a drug (for example, allergic reactions and gastro-intestinal bleeding from non-steroidal anti-inflammatory drugs). HALF OF THESE ADVERSE REACTIONS ARE PREVENTABLE! (*Sources – J.A.M.A., April 15, 1998; Prescriber's Newsletter, May, 1998.*)

167. Looking at the above statement, it would be prudent to note that if those patients who have GI bleeding take food supplements (for example: large doses of vitamin E or large doses of herbal supplements such as ginkgo, garlic, ginger, certain foods such as black tree fungus,) will have worse hemorrhaging than if they took no supplements.

168. "Unfortunately there are **too many in health care** who feel that if **it hasn't happened to them** the **adverse experiences of others do not apply**!" Part of the statement from Michael Cohen M.S. FASHP, President Institute of Safe Medications Practices. *Reported in Sentinel event alert - a Publication of JCAHO.*

169. Drug dosages should be reduced for the elderly and for renal failure patients. (Their bodies cannot handle drugs like healthy, normal people's bodies!)

170. Pre-labeled syringes should be aligned to the label on the medication ampule, and only then should the drug be drawn-up into the syringe. The drug administration should not proceed until after the patient's I.D. wrist band has been checked. If you are still not sure about the patient's name, ask him or her. [Pre-Aligned Injectate Method: PAI] (Don't be **distracted** when drawing up medications)

171. Early CPR (0-2 minutes), very early defibrillation (0-4 minutes) and ACLS (within 8 minutes of a patient with witnessed collapse of a ventricular fibrillation as the initial rhythm) produce 30 percent survival rate in contrast to no CPR and delayed defibrillation, in which case studies show there is a 0-2 percent rate of survival. – (ACLS Handbook for 1997-99, American Heart Association.)

NOTE: *All places for public gathering – such as stadiums, ball parks, transportation ter-*

62

*minals and airplanes – should have a working defibrillator and personnel trained to use it. It is **shocking to note** that many such places do not.*

172. Of the 40,684 heart attack admissions to Pennsylvania hospitals in 1993, risk-adjusted mortality was lower for patients treated by cardiologists, and patients thus treated had a lower mortality and shorter hospital stay. *(Nash et al, Journal of the American College of Cardiology, March, 1997)*

173. The Scandinavian Simvastatin Survival Study – looking at statins and heart disease – reported that patients **who gain weight** while on statins **derive** noticeably **less benefit** than those who lose or maintain body weight... only 19 percent vs. 38 percent cholesterol reduction.

174. Total mortality in middle-aged men is increased at low total cholesterol and LDL concentrations in smokers, but not in non-smokers. *(Cullen et al The Munster Heart Study (Procam) in Circulation 1997, Oct. 7, 96:2128-36)*

COMMENT: *This study shows that the deaths (mostly from lung cancer) were due to smok-*

ing, and not to the lowering of cholesterol. – Dr. Pai.

175. New research now underway in genetic therapy shows promise for reducing LDL cholesterol.

176. Raloxifene (Evista) decreases cardiovascular risk by reducing LDL cholesterol, lipoprotein (a), fibrinogen, and increasing HDL2-C without raising triglycerides in post-menopausal women. (*J.A.M.A., May 13, 1998*)

177. There is new evidence to suggest that **Raloxifene dramatically decreases breast cancer risk.** (*American Society of Clinical Oncologists, News Briefs from Annual Meeting, May 18, 1998*) (*However it increases clot formation*)

178. Cigar smokers have an increased incidence of **lung cancer** and also other forms of cancer. The risk of **mouth, esophagus and lip cancer is up tenfold.** Cigars also increase the risk of heart disease.

NOTE: *Cigars produce far more passive, or second-hand smoke than cigarettes, (University of California, Berkeley, Wellness Letter, June, 1998)*

COMMENT: *The radical surgery usually required for mouth and lip cancer caused by smoking or **chewing tobacco** can be quite disfiguring!*

179. Smoking has an adverse effect on **coronary artery disease in young women** —even those who **smoke only three to five cigarettes a day.** (*Johns Hopkins Medical Letter, Health After 50, June, 1998*)

COMMENT: **When somebody says "You've come a long way." They may be implying you've reached the end of the road. –Dr. Pai**

180. No amount of smoking is free of risk, according to the University of California, Berkeley, Wellness Letter. One may think he or she can control a light smoking habit, but eventually the habit controls the smoker!

181. Inactivity and lack of exercise by watching too much TV or "cruising the web" all the time, and a sedentary job, increases the risk of heart attack.

182. Losing as little as one and one half inches off the waistline reduced blood cholesterol significantly, according to the Tufts University Health & Nutrition Letter (*Oct., 1997*).

183. African Americans and Hispanic Americans are at greater risk of dying from a stroke at an early age than whites, according to a Texas study published in Stroke. *(Johns Hopkins Medical Letter Health After 50, August, 1997).*

184. Oral minoxidil can cause pericardial effusion, which is an uncommon but nonetheless serious complication. It can occur in patients with normal cardiovascular and renal function. Effusion usually clears when the drug is discontinued, but will recur if treatment with minoxidil is resumed. *(Reich, Gott, 1981)* Topical minoxidil, now being marketed for male pattern baldness, can cause measurable cardiovascular effects in some individuals. *(Leenen et al, 1988. Source: Goodman & Gilman's The Pharmacological Basis of Therapeutics, Ninth Ed., McGraw Hill, 1996)*

185. University of Kansas researchers reported in 1997 that, by their measurements, green tea is 100 percent more effective than vitamin C and 25 percent more effective than vitamin E at protecting cells from damage linked to cancer, heart disease and other illnesses. They also found that the antioxidant EGCG (epigallocatechin-3-gallate), in green tea, is twice as powerful as the antioxidant in red wine, grapes and other foods.

186. Green tea for skin cancer protection: Mice fed green tea and then exposed to ultra-violet light **had 94 percent fewer tumors** compared to the control group. But mice that were fed decaffeinated green tea had as many tumors as the control group, thus showing that the decaffeinated green tea offered no protection against skin cancer. (*American Health Foundation at Rutgers University*)

187. Adding milk to green tea neutralizes its health benefits.

188. Patients on coumadin should not take green tea.

189. Drinking one cup of green tea a week reduced esophageal cancer risk by 60 percent.

190. People **who drink burning-hot green tea** and **other boiling liquids** have a **five-fold increase in esophageal cancer** over those who do not. **Repeated thermal injury to the esophagus** may **increase cancer risk**. (*Source: National Cancer Insti-*

tute, U.S. and Shanghai Cancer Institute)

COMMENT: *This can be compared to Kashmiris who keep an earthen pot filled with glowing charcoal to keep them warm in winter. Over a period of time they develop cancer of the skin over the abdomen, which comes in contact with the earthen pot.*

Also, extremely high oral cancer risk has been observed in southeast Asians who smoke with the **lighted end** of the cigarette or mini-cigars (temperatures up to 600 degrees centigrade) **inside their mouths.**

COMMENT: *1. Candle in the windpipe - goodbye alveoli*

2. More tar and more waste with an utter lack of taste.

191. Soy protein, rather than animal protein, **significantly decreased total cholesterol,** LDL cholesterol and triglycerides. *(Cardiology, 1996)*

192. Heart attack patients in medicare pilot program get better treatment *(J.A.M.A., May 6, 1998)* The researchers believe that cooperative cardiovascular project *(established by a national panel of experts)* provides some evidence that quality improvement is achievable in today's environment of cost control.

193. Professional peers influence heart attack care options. *(J.A.M.A., May 6, 1998)*

194. High blood pressure increases the loss of brain cells with aging and the results in decline in the cognitive function. *(National Institute of Aging)*

195. Exercise keeps both the body and mind young. *(Dutch study in American College of Sports Medicine.)*

196. Death from strokes is increasing as Americans age. The National Stroke Association estimates that **730,000 Americans now suffer from stroke each year, and almost 160,000 people die from them.**

197. Supplementation with B-Carotene for 12 years was not associated with either benefit or harm with regards to mortality, incidence of malignancy or cardiovascular morbidity. *(N Eng J Med 1996, 334:1145-1149.)*

Supplementation of B-Carotene and Retinol for an average of **4 years in smokers and workers exposed to asbestos had an increase in incidence of lung cancer and mortality.** *(N Eng J Med 1996, 334:1150-1151.)*

198. Vitamin E (Tocopherol) Therapy in coronary artery disease patients reduced the rate of non fatal heart attacks. However there was no effect on cardiovascular mortality or total mortality.

199. Tirofiban (Aggrastat®) (anti-clotting protein in snake venom) when taken with aspirin and heparin reduced the likelihood of death and heart attack by 32 percent compared to treatment with aspirin and heparin alone. *Dr. Pierre Theroux and co-investigators at the Montreal Heart Institute (N. Eng J Med 1998; 338: 1488-1497.)*

200. Viagra® (Sildenafil) should not be prescribed for men taking nitrates, as this combination has additive hypotensive (low blood pressure) effects. *(Prescribers Newsletter, April, 1998.)*

COMMENT: – Erection Hypotension Syndrome? – Treatment: mast trousers with a no fly zone? – Dr. Pai.

201. On May 21, 1998 press release from Pfizer Headline News said that Nitroglycerin and Viagra® (Sildenafil) can cause severe, and fatal hypotension (low blood pressure) Pfizer said that patients on Viagra®

70

should not take nitroglycerin within 24 hours after taking Viagra®.

COMMENT: Currently there are more people on some form of nitroglycerin than on Viagra®. Nitroglycerin is a life saving drug — never stop any medication or start any medication without consulting your doctor.

202. Fatal drug interaction can occur between inhaled "poppers" (which are amyl or butyl nitrate which came in a glass ampule that needs to be popped open - These drugs supposedly enhance sex) and Viagra® *(Prescribers Newsletter June 1998)*

COMMENT: 1. These are non-cardiac patients on organic nitrates. 2. Patients may not tell the health care provider about illicit drug use. 3. No history may be available if the patient is nonresponsive.

203. As of June 10, 1998, sixteen deaths have been reported in patients on Viagra during or after sexual activity. Some of the patients were on nitroglycerin and others had bad cardiac disease. An FDA spokesman says "There is no direct link (between Viagra and the deaths), However we are going to continue to monitor these reports."

COMMENT: 1. There are no reports of how many men die during or after sex without Viagra. 2. Patients may need to take some type of stress test if they plan to have sex after years of sexual inactivity.

204. Primary prevention of acute coronary events with Lovastatin in men and women with average cholesterol levels. (*Downs et al J.A.M.A., 1998; 279: 1615-1622 May 27, 1998*)

Lovastatin reduces the risk for the acute major coronary event in men and women with average total cholesterol and LDL cholesterol levels and below average HDL cholesterol levels.

Implications of this study:

1. HDL cholesterol - low level is a risk factor.

2. Reassessment of National Cholesterol Education Program Guidelines regarding pharmacological intervention.

3. Approximately **6 million** Americans currently not recommended for drug treatment **may benefit** from LDL-C reduction with Lovastatin.

205. Antiatherothrombotic properties of statins.

Implications of cardiovascular event reduction. (*Rosenson and Tangney J.A.M.A., 1998; 279: 1643-1650 May 27, 1998*)

The beneficial effects of statins on clinical events may involve nonlipid mechanisms **that modify endothelial function, inflammatory responses, plaque stability and thrombus formation.**

Experimental animal models suggest: Statins decrease macrophages and decrease cholesterol ester content and increase the volume of collagen and smooth muscle cells. Statins mitigate the thrombotic sequence of plaque disruption through inhibition of platelet aggregation and maintenance of a favorable balance between prothrombotic sequence of plaque disruption through inhibition of platelet aggregation and maintenance of a favorable balance between prothrombotic and fibrinolytic mechanisms.

These nonlipid properties of statins may help to **explain the early and significant cardiovascular event reduction reported in several clinical trials of statin therapy.**

206. Postmenopausal hormonal use and risk of colorectal cancer and adenoma (*Francine Grodstien et al of Brigham and Women's Hospital and Harvard Medical School of Public Health Annuals of Inter Med, May 1, 1998; 128: 705-712*) In this large prospective study, **the risk of colon and rectal cancers was decreased by 35% among women currently using postmenopausal hormone replacement therapy.**

207. Cancer Prevention: Better late than never? (*Editorial: Annals of Inter Medicine, May 1, 1998; 128: 771-772.*) This article discusses several studies associated with different carcinogens and cancer prevention. One interesting statement in this article states that detailed studies of cigarette smokers revealed **meaningful declines in the risk for lung and bladder cancer within a few years of smoking cessation,** even among people who **smoked hundreds of thousands of cigarettes.**

208. Association between multiple cardiovascular risk factors and atherosclerosis in children and young adults.
G. Berenson, M.D. S. Srinivansan, Ph.D.

and Co-workers, for the Bogalusa Heart Study (*N Eng J Med, June 4, 1998; 338: 1650-1656*)

This study was done because of the limited information available on the relationship between multiple risk factors and asymptomatic atherosclerosis in young people. Autopsies were done on **204 young persons ages 2 to 39 who had died from different causes but principally trauma.** Data was on antemortem risk factors was available on **93** of these persons who were the focus of the study.

The conclusions from the study was that **as the cardiovascular risk factors increases so does the severity of asymptomatic coronary and aortic atherosclerosis in young people.**

COMMENT: *Worst offenders accelerating atherosclerosis in young people*

1. Cigarette smoking – especially in young people with other risk factors

2. Obesity

3. High cholesterol

4. Glycosylated Hemoglobin (from sustained high blood sugar)

209. When should heart disease prevention begin? *(Editorial by J. Michael Gaziano, M.D., M.P.H. Harvard medical school. N Eng J Med, June 4, 1998; 338: 1690-1692)* Editorial discusses various studies on atherosclerosis, risk factors, autopsy studies and public health issues.

One interesting statement in this article is that **most adolescents value plans for next Saturday night** more than their **quality of life in the sixth or seventh decade.**

210. Reversing heart disease: **Rating the different diets.** *(The Johns Hopkins Medical Letter after 50 May 1997)*

211. Cigarette smoking causes **hearing loss** *(J.A.M.A., News June 3, 1998)* COMMENT: *Wife complaining about husband - no matter how much I ask him to quit smoking he never **listens** to me.*

212. Cigarette smoking during pregnancy causes more damage to the fetal brain (affects behavior and learning) than cocaine addiction.

213. Non-smokers who live with heavy smokers are four times as likely to have

heart attacks than those who live in smoke free households. Fourteen percent of the heart attacks in men and 18% of those in women could be attributed to **passive smoking**. Non-smokers had a **59% increase** in heart attacks when they lived with a spouse who smoked. *Research from Argentinian hospitals.*

214. Pathophysiology of **sudden coronary death in women** - implications on prevention (*Suzanne Oparil M.D. Univ of Al at Birmingham Circulation 1998; 97: 2103-2105*)

In this article Dr. Oparil says that in one epidemiological study **cigarette smoking was the strongest risk factor for sudden cardiac death among women**. The most common lesion found in cigarette smokers in the Burke study was **plaque erosion**.

215. More Heart attacks in winter - 53% more cases of heart attacks were reported in the winter months than in summer. (*Spencer f. et al J Am Coll Cardiology.May 1998 31: 1266-33*)

216. Acute respiratory tract infections and (increased) risk of first time Acute M.I. (heart attack) in people without a history of clinical risk factors for A.M.I. Acute respiratory tract infections (colds) were associated with an increased risk of A.M.I. for a period of two weeks. *E. Meier, Christopher R. Lancet 351: 1467-71 (May 16, 1998)*

Possible Mechanisms -

Increased C-Reactive protein

Systemic inflammation

Altered endothelial function - causing plaque rupture, changes in clotting factors such as fibrinogen, increase in inflammatory cytokines which inhibit vasodilating nitric oxide or prostaglandins.

Limitation of the study: The common cold picture itself may have been an early symptom of the heart attack.

COMMENT: Another good reason to take aspirin and antioxidants during a cold (for adults) -Dr. Pai.

217. Effect of lowering average or below average cholesterol levels on the progression of carotid atherosclerosis

*CONCLUSIONS: **Treatment with pravastatin (Pravachol®) reduced the development of carotid atherosclerosis among patients***

with **coronary heart disease** and a wide range of pretreatment cholesterol levels. Treatment with this agent **prevented** any detectable increase in **carotid wall thickening** over **four years of follow up**. (*Circulation 1998; 97: 1784-1799 May 12, 1998*)

218. Prediction of coronary heart disease using risk factor categories. (*Peter W.F. Wilson et al Circulation 1998; 97: 1837-1847 May 12, 1998*). In this study the prediction algorithms have been adapted to simplified score sheets that allow physicians to estimate multivariate CHD risk in middle aged patients.

219. Plasma C-Reactive protein and the risk of developing peripheral vascular disease. (*Circulation 1998; 425-428*) *Paul M. Ridker M.D. et al* The data obtained from this study indicate that among **apparently healthy men**, baseline levels of C-Reactive protein predict future risk of developing peripheral arterial disease and thus provide further support for the hypotheses that the chronic inflammation is important in the pathogenies of atherothrombosis.

COMMENT: *C-Reactive protein which is a marker for systemic inflammation has al-*

ready been implicated in heart attacks and thromboembolic strokes in apparently healthy men. Remember that cardiovascular disease affects 65 miles of arteries.

220. New rules for high blood pressure - Cardiovascular News, *(Ruth Sorelle Circulation News writer Circulation 1998; 97: 307-308 Feb 3 1998)* In it's sixth report from the joint national committee on prevention, detection, evaluation and treatment of high blood pressure: **1.** 75% with high blood pressure do not have it controlled. **2.** 25% with high blood pressure have controlled their blood pressure. **3.** 25% are on medication but not controlled. **4.** 50% of the patients are not on medications at all. This according to Dr. Sheldon G. Sheps, M.D. Emeritus Professor of Medicine at the Mayo Clinic in Rochester, Minn., The chairman of the joint National Committee on Prevention, Detection, Evaluation and Treatment of High Blood Pressure. According to Keith Ferdinand M.D. of Heartbeats Life Center in New Orleans, African Americans with high rates of high blood pressure also have more end stage renal disease, stroke and myocardial infarction.

The main message we want to get out is "Get your blood pressure controlled," and "Don't be satisfied if your blood pressure is not controlled." said Dr. Sheps.

COMMENT: Some patients may need a higher dose or a different drug or a combination of drugs to bring their blood pressure to normal.

221. The Hypertension Optimal Treatment Study which involved 18,790 patients from 26 countries over 5 years concluded that

1. Diastolic blood pressure to 83 mm of Hg) reduced the heart attack rate 37% compared to those at a diastolic pressure of 90.

2. Among patients with preexisting coronary artery disease when their diastolic blood pressure was reduced to 80 (mm of Hg) this group of patients had 43% fewer strokes.

3. 75 mg of aspirin (80mg = baby aspirin and 325mg = regular adult tablet) reduced the heart attack rate significantly.

4. Even though the optimal blood pressure is 120 (systolic) / 80 (diastolic) 50 million Americans have blood pressures greater than

140/90. and that hypertension contributes to nearly one million heart attacks a year.

COMMENT: *In hypertension the hydrostatic pressure in the blood drives the low density cholesterol from the blood into the arterial vessel wall. Uncontrolled hypertension can cause end organ dysfunction of the brain, heart and kidneys. Hypertension shrinks the brain (causes loss of brain tissue), increases strokes, causes increased thickness of the heart muscle (left ventricular hypertrophy) increases coronary artery disease (increasing the demand for oxygen and concomitantly decreasing the supply of oxygen.) Hypertension also causes kidney failure.*

222. American Heart Association Call to Action **obesity as a major risk factor for coronary disease.** Robert H. Ecker M.D. Ronald M. Krauss M.D. for the AHA Nutrition Committee (*Circulation, 1998; 97: 2099-2100*)

223. Abdominal fat content has been implicated as a risk for cardiovascular disease. Low fat, low calorie diet with exercise reduces the waist size, decreasing the cardiovascular risk.

COMMENT: The waist is a terrible thing to life - Dr. Pai

224. Garlic lowers LDL cholesterol (bad cholesterol), inhibits platelet aggregation, and stimulates fibrinolytic activity. (*Dr. Donald Hensrud – Mayo Clinic Teleconference, March 21, 1998.*)

225. Garlic oil in experimental atherosclerosis. (*Letter to the Editor, LANCET, April 24, 1976.*) Garlic oil reversed atherosclerosis.

226. Onion and garlic in experimental atherosclerosis; *Dr. R.C. Jain; May 31, 1975; Letter to the Editor, LANCET;* Garlic reversed atherosclerosis; onion did not. (Note - Onion and garlic when discussed in the medical community raise a stink. The formulations are not standardized in the U.S.) Standardization is good in Germany. However, remember, too much garlic intake can cause bleeding.

227. Spontaneous **spinal epidural hematoma** (blood clot) with associated platelet dysfunction from **excessive garlic ingestion**: A Case Report (*Dr. Ken D. Rose, Dept. of Surgery, Pontiac General Hospital, in Neurosurgery 26:880-882, 1990.*)

228. Effect of garlic oil preparation on serum lipoproteins and cholesterol metabolism. *Heiner K. Berthold, M.D. P.H.D. et al J.A.M.A., June, 17, 1998; 1900-1902.*

The **commercial garlic oil** preparation **had no influence** on serum lipoproteins, cholesterol absorption or cholesterol synthesis. Garlic therapy for treatment of hypercholesterolemia cannot be recommended on the basis of this study. (*German Study*)

229. An experimental model of sudden death due to low energy chest wall impact (Commotio Cordis) *N Eng J Med, June 18, 1998; 338: 1805-11 M.S. Link M.D. et al*

Fatal Impact- Concussion of the Heart. Gregory D Curfman M.D. *editorial N Eng J Med 1998; 338: 1841-1843*

The above article and the editorial explain how low impact injury to the left chest wall with a baseball or a hockey puck could result in "Commotio Cordis" (or concussion of the heart,) in many young people who died due to ventricular fibrillation as they could not be resuscitated.

COMMENT: Wear chest protection or use safety baseballs.

230. Helicobacter Pylori strains and Ischemic Heart Disease. *Vincenzo Pasceri, M.D. et al*

Patients with ischemic heart disease had a higher prevalence of cytotoxin - associated gene - a positive strain of Helicobacter Pylori. Virulent H Pylori may influence atherogenesis through low grade persistent inflammatory stimulation. (*Circulation May 5, 1998; 97: 1675-1679*)

COMMENT: 1. We thought in the past that H. Pylori cause only peptic ulcers, now we have a ulcer - heart disease link previously attributed only to type A personality. 2. H. Pylori are spread by house flies. - Dr. Pai

231. Prolongation of the QT interval and sudden infant death syndrome. *N Eng J Med, June 11, 1998; 1709-1714* Prolongation of QT interval in the first week of life is strongly associated with SIDS. Neonatal EKG recommended for infants at risk.

232. Too much coffee raises the stroke risk in older men with hypertension.
COMMENT: There was an older study which showed that one cup of coffee could raise the systolic blood pressure by as much as 10mm of mercury.

233. Research at Harvard Medical school revealed that a large number of the 7,000 patients in the US and Canada are not filling their prescriptions for cholesterol lowering drugs, putting themselves at a increased risk of heart attack, strokes and premature death. *Tufts University Health E Nutrition Letter, July 1998*

234. The migraine drugs Sumitriptan and Dihydroergotamine (DHE Nasal Spray) can cause blood vessels to constrict and may be harmful to people with Coronary Artery Disease.

235. American Heart Association call to action - Obesity as a major risk factor for coronary disease. *Robert H. Eckel M.D., Ronald M. Krauss M.D. for the AHA Nutrition Committee (Circulation, 1998; 97: 2099-2100)* The N.I.H. decreased the weight at which people are determined to be obese or overweight. This determination takes into account the actual weight and body mass index rather than the fat content of the body (now even muscular people can fall into this category). The full report is to be released at the end of June 1998. Overnight 29 million

Americans are in the overweight category. The guidelines propose using the body mass index or the BMI to assess patients correlates to body weight, mostly to body fat except in very muscular persons. The pre-1995 federal guidelines identified BMI of 27.8 for men and 27.3 for women. The 1995 guidelines defined overweight as BMI of 25-29 and obesity as BMI of 30 or more. Health risks start increasing at a BMI of 25.

American Heart Association recommends weight loss if patients have a BMI of 27 or more with two or more risk factors and a waist circumference of greater than 35 inches in women and 40 inches in men. The new BMI is the same standard used in Europe. American Heart Association recommends six months of non drug therapy and subsequent drug therapy with diet and exercise.

*COMMENT: No Pain, No {Weight} Loss! Time for more diet and exercise. Exercise caution with exercise. There are many fitness buffs in the emergency rooms and in the operating rooms. Beware of **girth control** pills.*

236. New N.I.H. Guidelines recommend people to lose 10% body weight when the BMI exceeds 25.

237. Ideal body weight (kilos) = height in centimeters - 100.

Ideal body weight in kg=cm-100.

note: 1 meter = 100cm; 1 kg = 2.204 lbs. 1 inch = 2.540 cm.

*NOTE: Always consult your **doctor and pharmacist before using a new drug**, nutritional supplement or exercise regimen. Your doctor should always be kept aware of your food habits, medication and supplement intake.*

Weigh the FA(c)Ts

body mass index: BMI= $\dfrac{703 \times \text{Weight in Pounds}}{(\text{Height in Inches})^2}$ BMI= $\dfrac{\text{Weight in Kilos}}{(\text{Height in Meters})^2}$ 1 kilo=2.204lbs 1in=2.540cm

	Body Mass Index measured by height and weight				Previously healthy; now overweight		In old standard, woman overweight at 27, men at 28			Obese		(BMI above 35) Morbid Obesity	
	21	22	23	24	25	26	27	28	29	30	31	35	36
5'	107	112	118	123	128	133	138	143	138	153	158	179.5	184.5
5'1"	111	116	122	127	132	137	143	148	153	158	164	185.5	191
5'3"	118	124	130	135	141	146	152	158	163	169	175	198	203.5
5'5"	126	132	138	144	150	156	162	168	174	180	185	210.5	216.5
5'7"	134	140	146	153	159	166	172	178	185	191	198	224	230
5'9"	142	149	155	162	169	176	182	189	196	203	209	237.5	244
5'11"	150	157	165	172	179	186	193	200	208	215	222	251	258.5
6'1"	159	166	174	182	189	197	204	212	219	227	235	266	273
6'3"	168	176	184	192	200	208	216	224	232	240	248	280.5	288.2
					29 million adults		29 million adults			25 million adults		14 million adults	

Overweight, obesity, morbid obesity: increased risk of cardiovascular disease and cancer. Patients with morbid obesity have twice the perioperative morbidity and mortality owing to the associated cardiovascular respiratiory abnormalities and hypercoagulability. Chart modified from National Center for Health Statistics data.

NON CARDIAC NEW DEVELOPMENTS

1. A pheromone receptor was recently found in the human nose. 30 years back Martha McClintock noticed that the menstrual cycle of women living together tended to synchronize over time. A new modality of communication has been discovered something beyond sight, sound, taste, scent and touch; human pheromones -Journal Watch Audio Vol 9 Number 8 - April 15, 1998

2. **Drug stops compulsive buying.** A University of Iowa study found that fluvuxamine (Luvox, Solvay-Upjohn) boosted sales resistance by at least half for nine out of ten compulsive shoppers. In the open label study; there were significant reductions in shopping frequency and the amount of money spent. One man dropped his clothing purchases from $800 to $200 a month. Dr. Donald Blacks presentation to American Psychiatric Association reported in Physicians weekly July 17, 1995

COMMENT: watch for a drug induced recession. -Dr. Pai

CARDIAC RISK FACTORS:
Something within your control to modify

1. **Tobacco** Smoking *active and passive*
2. **High LDL** ("Bad Cholesterol!")
3. **High Triglycerides**
4. **Small dense LDL**
5. Low HDL ("Good Cholesterol")
6. Lipoprotein APO B
7. Lipoprotein A [LP(a)] (difficult to treat)
8. IDL
9. **Diabetes Mellitus**
10. **High Blood Pressure**
11. **Obesity**
12. Fasting Hyperinsulinemia
13. Chlamydia
14. Gingivitis
15. Homocysteine
16. Stress
17. Fibrinogen
18. Increased Iron
19. Post-menopausal Women (Hormone Replacement Therapy can modify this risk factor!) New controversy, HRT increases risk in the first year. No reduction in risk up to 4.1 years, and reduces risk after several years of therapy *(Modified from J.A.M.A. Aug 19, 1998, 280 605-613)*

20. Lack of Regular Meaningful Exercise
21. Impaired glucose tolerance
22. Hyperuricemia
23. Gout
24. Oral contraceptive use
25. High - C-reactive protein
26. High plasminogen activation inhibitor
27. Interleukin-2
28. Increased SICAM-1 level (above 75th percentile)
29. Mercury
30. Air pollution
31. Cocaine
32. Anger (in up to 25% of the sudden death from any cardiac cause.)
33. Hostility
34. New onset depression in men.
35. Increased plasma viscosity.

CARDIAC RISK FACTORS: Beyond Our Control

1. **Male gender**
2. **Family History** of CAD before 55
3. **Increasing Age**
4. Race *(increased incidence among the Asian-Indians, Pakistanis, Bangladeshis and whites) (Asian Indian incidence is four times more than whites)*
   5. Low birth weight
   6. Ear lobe crease

MEDICAL HISTORY CHECKLIST

for

_____
(Your name goes here)

Patient No. _ _ _ _ _ _ _

Gender: ☐ Male   ☐ Female

Age: _____ Years   Height _____ in.
Weight _____ lbs

Date of Most Recent Physical Exam: _____

VITAL STATISTICS

(It is vital to keep the numbers in the normal range so that you don't become a statistic!)

Brief personal clinical history, including risk factor for Cardiovascular Disease:

☐ History of Heart Disease
☐ Stroke
☐ Peripheral Vascular Disease
☐ History of Diabetes
☐ Hypertension
☐ History of cardiac or vascular surgery

☐ Smoking - **Active and passive**
　　Past and present and
　　quantity and duration

Beer drinking:
☐ 1 - 2 bottles/day (12-24 oz)
☐ More than 3 bottles at one time
Red wine consumption:
☐ Other alcohol - specify type and
　　quantity per day
Coffee type, quantity
Tea type, quantity
· Green tea consumption, quantity

Drug Abuse:

　　Type: _____

　　Quantity: _____

☐ Obesity
☐ Family History of Heart Disease

Medications (ask your doctor or pharmacist)

☐ Ace Inhibitors
☐ Angiotensin-II receptor blockers
☐ Beta Blockers
☐ Calcium Channel Blocker

Diuretics:

- [ ] Thiazide
- [ ] Triamterene
- [ ] Loop Diuretics
- [ ] Spironolactone
- [ ] Amiloride

Other Medications:

- [ ] Cholesterol-lowering Drugs
- [ ] Vitamins and food supplements

Clinical Data:

- [ ] Systolic Blood Pressure: _____
- [ ] Diastolic Blood Pressure _____
- [ ] Heart Rate _____
- [ ] Body Mass Index _____
- [ ] Waist circumference _____
- [ ] Hip Height-Height Ratio _____
- [ ] Waist Hip Ratio _____
- [ ] Presence of truncal obesity _____
- [ ] Ear lobe crease _____
- [ ] Male Pattern Baldness _____

DIETARY REGIMEN:

This checklist is for your use in preparing for a physical exam by your family physician. It is important that you give your physician accurate and truthful information so you can derive the greatest benefit from the exam.

Vegetarian:

Quantity and Type of Fiber Intake
_____ *grams/day*
_____ Actual fruit and vegetable intake

Quantity and Type of Fat Intake
Saturated _____ *grams/day*
Monounsaturated _____ *grams/day*
Polyunsaturated _____ *grams/day*

Non Vegetarian
Quantity of meat intake
Quantity and type of fat intake
Use of trans fats - Quantity (margarines)
Intake of fatty fish or other types of fish
Intake of salads, fresh fruits and vegetables
Intake of supplemental fiber
Intake of Sitostanol (Pine Margarine)
Intake of refined sugars
Pastries and "sugary" Fats

LAB TESTS:

- ☐ Hemoglobin _____
- ☐ Hematocrit _____
- ☐ Total White Cell count _____
- ☐ EKG _____
- ☐ Differential count: _____
- ☐ Polys _____ Lymphocytes _____
- ☐ Basophils _____
- ☐ Eosinophils _____
- ☐ Na _____
- ☐ K _____
- ☐ Magnesium _____
- ☐ CL _____
- ☐ Fasting Blood Glucose _____
- ☐ Blood urea _____
- ☐ Serum creatinine _____
- ☐ Serum Uric Acid _____
- ☐ Serum bilirubin _____
- ☐ SGOT _____
- ☐ SGPT _____
- ☐ GGT _____
- ☐ Serum CK _____
- ☐ CKMB _____
- ☐ Total Cholesterol: _____
- ☐ LDL, _____
- ☐ HDL _____

- [ ] LP (a) _____
- [ ] Fasting Triglycerides _____
- [ ] Bleeding Time _____

(preferably before and after aspirin therapy - Bleeding times may be prolonged by garlic, Ginkgo biloba, black tree fungus, large doses of vitamin E and anti-inflammatory agents.)

ADDITIONAL TESTS:

- [ ] Fasting serum insulin
- [ ] 2 H Post oral GTT Glucose
- [ ] Homocysteine Level
- [ ] Folate level
- [ ] Serum B-12 *(to avoid masking B-12 Deficiency with Folic Acid)*
- [ ] Serum Iron
- [ ] Serum C - Reactive Protein
- [ ] Fibrinogen level
- [ ] PAI Level
- [ ] Soluble intercellular adhesion molecule-1 level
- [ ] APO B level
- [ ] Small, dense LDL level
- [ ] IDL
- [ ] Immunologic tests for previous chlamydia infection

- [ ] New, non-invasive chlamydia testing using urine sample
- [ ] HBA1C (Shows glycemic control – Shows **how long the cherries** (RBC's) **have been in the sugar syrup** (hyperglycemic blood).)

Exercise/Stress Reduction/Behavior

Exercise: Type, frequency, intensity

Behavior, Personality

Frequency of Verbal Conflicts

Episodes of anger/ week

Feelings of helplessness

Sense of impending doom

Frustration

Stress reduction

Medication/Supplements: Type, Duration *(Keep a record of the Chronology of Intake of medications, supplements and foods)*

Breathing exercise

Stretch exercise like yoga and Tai-chi (Check with your doctor first! Some of the exercises – like standing on your neck and head – may not be for everyone!)

Blood pressure and heart rate measurement before and after stress reduction therapy

Risk factor reduction for heart disease should not fizzle-out like New Year's resolutions. **Patients should measure their progress one day at a time.** The patient should keep a record of "heart-friendly" and "heart-hostile" deeds he or she has done each day. If more "heart-friendly" activity is performed, such as eating a heart-healthy meal, good exercise, stress reduction, intake of vitamin E, folic acid, vitamins B-6 and B-12, vitamin C, a relaxed day at work, home, school, or a social gathering, mark the day as a **Good Heart Day** (or a Good Artery Day). Examples of a **Bad Heart Day** (or a Bad Artery Day) include: a "bad day" at work, home, or school; a 2- or 3-pack cigarette day; a day of more than three beers at one session; a day of high-fat meals that included fatty meats and/or trans-fat pastries; a day of living or working in a polluted environment; and a day of uncontrolled or untreated diabetes or hypertension.

It is a good idea to keep a **daily log of "Good Heart Days" and "Bad Heart Days," on a 3x5 index card for yourself** for motivation, and every few months you can show your doctor the positive or negative changes in your lifestyle.

**Remember it's vital
not to become a statistic!**™

1. Cardiovascular disease kills more Americans than cancer, AIDS, all types of accidents, suicides and homicides combined.
   TRUE

2. Heart Disease is the No. 1 killer of American women.
   TRUE

3. Heart Disease kills more women than men.
   TRUE

4. The process of atherosclerosis (fatty buildup within the arteries) starts as early as age two years.
   TRUE

5. Homocysteine is responsible for about ten percent of all cardiovascular deaths.
   TRUE

6. Chlamydia — a sexually-transmitted disease — may cause coronary artery disease.
   TRUE

7. Gingivitis (periodontal gum disease)

may contribute to heart disease.
TRUE

8. Moderate alcoholic beverage intake can decrease the risk of heart disease.
TRUE

9. Beer bingeing is associated with increased heart disease.
TRUE

10. There are adequate preventive cardiology services to handle the epidemic of heart disease.
FALSE

11. Cholesterol lowering statins have more benefits than just lowering cholesterol.
TRUE

12. A person with a normal EKG, echocardiogram and stress test can still have a heart attack without warning.
TRUE

13. Lowering cholesterol levels even in normal people protects against cardiovascular disease.
TRUE

14. Saturated fat content of the food is more important than the cholesterol content in raising blood cholesterol.
TRUE

The typical Western diet and lifestyle is a fertilizer for cancer and cardiovascular disease. – *Dr. Pai*

TYPICAL WESTERN DIET AND LIFESTYLE:

Lack of exercise with weight gain
+ High body iron stores + Isolation
High Fat + Red Meat + Stress + Smoking
(accelerate both cancer and cardiovascular disease!)

Effect On

Atherosclerotic Cardiovascular Disease	→ Atherosclerotic Cardiovascular Disease	→ Atherosclerotic Cardiovascular Disease	→ Atherosclerotic Cardiovascular Disease	→ Atherosclerotic Cardiovascular Disease
Cancer	→ Cancer	→ Cancer	→ Cancer	Cancer

(DEATH)

Chart by Dr. Pai

104

SWITCHING TO A LOW-FAT, HIGH FIBER VEGETARIAN DIET + STOP SMOKING

Social or Community Support Groups

With Stress Reduction, Exercise with Weight Loss + Certain Antioxidants Can Reduce/Reverse/Prevent Cardiovascular Disease and Decrease Cancer Risk!

Effect On

Cancer Risk	←	Atherosclerotic Cardiovascular Disease
Cancer Risk	←	Atherosclerotic Cardiovascular Disease
Cancer Risk	←	Atherosclerotic Cardiovascular Disease
Cancer Risk	←	Atherosclerotic Cardiovascular Disease

Chart by Dr. Pai
105

Copyright © 1998 Dr. Pai

TYPICAL WESTERN DIET AND LIFESTYLE

High Fat + Red Meat + Stress + Smoking

Effect On

Atherosclerotic Cardiovascular Disease
Cholesterol-Lowering Statins

➡️

Atherosclerotic Cardiovascular Disease

➡️

Atherosclerotic Cardiovascular Disease

➡️

Stopped Or Reversed By Cholesterol-Lowering Statins

Cancer ➡️ Cancer ➡️ Cancer ➡️ ## Cancer
Growth Goes Unchecked

Chart by Dr. Pai

106

I recently was discussing prevention and reversal of heart disease with a colleague who said, "Ultimately, everyone has to die." My point is this: untimely death is to be prevented; as for ultimately — no one is sure what ultimately is because of the effect of the new cholesterol-lowering drugs on the actual increase in life span.

To use Wall Street jargon, just as the value of an investment is compounded with time, so is the growth of a plaque in the human circulatory system. The more risk factors the patient is subjected to the more aggressive is the progress of the growth of the plaque. Risk factor modification should be the first priority.

Diet and exercise help, but in sedentary patient with severe coronary artery disease and unstable plaque, heavy snow shoveling and unaccustomed exercise during hunting expeditions can cause a heart attack.

For a person with coronary artery disease **the most difficult transition is from "it can never happen to me" to "why me?"** Remember that all is not lost — with risk factor modification, cholesterol-lowering medications and supplements, coronary artery disease can be reversed.

Drug therapy should be considered early because diet and exercise fail in a vast majority of people. In a study of patients with identical cholesterol levels – one group on statin treatment and another without statin treatment – patients on statin treatment had fever cardiovascular events. The statin drugs do have side effects but their benefits outweigh the risks.

Hormone replacement therapy (HRT) (New controversy see page 91) not only decreases coronary artery disease and strengthens bone, but corrects the loss of balance associated with aging by the effects of the hormones on the neuromuscular system and **prevents falls** that could cause fracture. HRT delays wrinkling of the skin. HRT, in older studies with larger doses, showed an increase in cancer incidence. But with these new **S.E.R.M.S. (selective estrogen receptor modulators** – smart estrogens), such as Raloxifene, there has been no increase in incidence of breast or uterine cancer. Raloxifene **dramatically reduces breast**

cancer risk. Estrogen therapy is related to its effect on nitric oxide production, which prevents oxidation of LDL-C, prevents smooth-muscle proliferation, prevents platelet aggregation, prevents inflammatory changes in smooth-muscle and promotes vasodilation. Raloxifene does not prevent hot flashes. Soy protein prevents hot flashes because they contain phytoestrogens. Soy protein also decreases breast cancer risk. HRT has now been shown to decrease colon cancer and improve blood sugar control in type 2 diabetes.

As with food and drinks, moderation is the key. If a total calorie restriction is implemented after full growth is achieved (after age 21) life span increases dramatically.

Eating a large quantity of high-calorie diet, low-fat food may be as bad as consuming a high-fat diet.

Consuming only small quantities of mustard as a condiment may not be hazardous, but the consumption of large quantities of mustard oil causes problems in the cardiac conduction system.

As for alcohol, there is an old saying in France: "There are more old drunkards than old doctors." This old saying was good in the olden days – even if the driver of the carriage was drunk the sober horses took him home. The French are known to consume more wine than any other type of alcohol, and mostly red wine.

Investigations of the recent Parisian tragedy in which the British Princess Diana died in a car crash suggested that excessive use of alcohol was one of the contributing factors. Through moderate alcohol use decreases the risk of heart disease it increases the risk of cancer.

To summarize a few highly important points:

- Stress reduction therapy is a must.
- Quitting smoking will definitely help.
- Control of diabetes and hypertension.
- The United States has one of the best interventional cardiac care systems, but has no effective preventive cardiac care. I have discussed this compatible cyclical cardiac regimen with many health institutions in the U.S. and abroad, and am in the process of

conducting research to prevent and reverse heart disease. In future years we will see this type of treatment with cholesterol-lowering drugs, food supplements, antibiotics, genetic engineering, control of risk factors and stress reduction therapy being used more often.

Some of the studies may contradict other studies, this happens occasionally in medical literature.

I coined the word Atherolysis™ over 25 years ago to designate my program for the prevention and reversal of heart disease.

I hope to be around to write some more updates to this book and I am confident that, if you take this information to heart, you will be around to read them.

Narendra M. Pai, M.D.
Lewistown, Pennsylvania

Comments: **1.** HRT Controversy page 91 pt. 19, applies to women with existing heart disease and not for healthy women. **2.** Folic acid prevents colon cancer (Nurses Health Study) and folic acid with B12 may reduce the risk of Alzheimers Disease (British Study). **3.** High resolution M.R.I show vulnerable plaques (A.H.A. 1998.)

FIRST HEART ATTACK RISK TEST

☐ **Age: Men**
0pts	Less than 35	**3pts**	49 to 53
1pts	35 to 39	**4pts**	54+
2pts	40 to 48		

Age: Female
0pts	Less than 42	**3pts**	55 to 73
1pts	42 to 44	**4pts**	74+
2pts	45 to 54		

☐ **Family History**
2 pts My family has a history of heart disease or heart attacks before the age of 60

☐ **Inactive Lifestyle**
1pt I rarely exercise or do anything physically demanding

☐ **Weight**
1pt I'm more than 20 lbs over my ideal weight

☐ **Smoking**
1pt I'm a smoker

☐ **Diabetic:**
1pt Male Diabetic
2pts Female Diabetic

☐ **Total Cholesterol Level**
0pt Less than 240 mg/dl
1pt 240 to 315 mg/dl
2pts More than 315 mg/dl

☐ HDL Level (good cholesterol)

0pts 39 to 59 mg/dl
1pt 30 to 38 mg/dl
2pts Under 30 mg/dl
-1pt Over 60 mg/dl

☐ Blood Pressure

I don't take blood pressure medication; my blood pressure is:

(Use your top or higher blood pressure number)

0pts Less than 140 mmHg
1pt 140 to 170 mmHg
2pts Greater than 170 mmHg

(or)

1pt I am currently taking blood pressure medication

☐ Total Points

If you scored 4 points or more, you could be at above average risk of a first heart attack compared to the general adult population. The more points you score, the greater your risk.

If you have already had a heart attack or have heart disease, your heart attack risk is significantly higher. Only your doctor can evaluate your risk and recommend treatment plans to reduce your risk. If you don't know your cholesterol level or blood pressure, ask your doctor if your levels should be checked.

Reprinted with permission of Bristol-Myers Squibb Company.

113

COMMENTS:

1. People who have a family history of heart disease, are inactive, smoke cigarettes, eat large quantities of red meat and saturated fat (...what I would call "mean cuisine"), and binge on beer, have high blood pressure, diabetes or syndrome X have the highest incidence of heart disease.

2. Negative life style changes shorten the life span.

3. Could reversal of renal artery atherosclerosis stop reno-vascular hypertension?

4. Could reversal of pudendal atherosclerosis cure impotence?

5. Looking at the effects of atherosclerosis reversal on stroke and heart attacks, this may also be beneficial to patients with peripheral vascular disease, preventing many limb ischemia amputations.

6. During cardio-pulmonary resuscitation (CPR) and ACLS in a cardiac arrest victim, a **pressurized I.V. bag** would probably be more effective in delivering drugs to the central circulation and heart than the traditional (non-pressurized) I.V. (Reason: Sometimes we see the hemodynamic effects of drugs given several minutes prior — immediately after the patient on femoral to femoral bypass — because the drug is rapidly delivered to the central circulation.)

7. A type of diabetes (Type III) that occurs widely in the Indian state of Kerala is attributed to excessive intake of tapioca, which supposedly contains a form of cyanide, which affects the pancreas.

8. Yoga stretch exercises— stretch the muscles all over the body thus:

a Increases the blood supply to the muscles. (need thermographic studies.)

b Decreases resistance to blood flow. (decreases the systemic vascular resistance thus decreases the workload on the heart and temporarily decrease blood pressure.)

c Increase the initial length of the muscle fiber — therefore increase the force of contraction (Starling's Law.) Studies are needed to measure the effect of yoga on blood glucose, lipid levels, blood lactate and the magnitude, direction and duration of blood pressure control and yogic effect on metabolism.

9. Yogic breathing exercises improve oxygenation of the blood by abolishing the oxygen/

blood. (V/Q) flow mixing mismatch (*Dr. Dean Ornish*).

10. Is non alcoholic red wine beneficial? New wine has more antioxidants than old wine.

11. One of the wines with a lot of antioxidants is Petit Sirah.

12. Accessibility to exercise machines in highway rest areas, airports and convention centers.

13. Does rapid lowering of cholesterol make patients anxious, argumentative and irritable?

14. Would intravenous Ketorolac be more effective than oral aspirin in preventing a clot formation after plaque rupture?

15. Would supplemental folic acid + B12 decrease neural canal deformity in the offspring of operating personnel? (Counteracts the effects of nitrous oxide pollution.)

16. Alpha Lipoic acid - a powerful antioxidant - both water and fat soluble decreases blood glucose. (Prescribed in Germany for Diabetic Neuropathy.)

17. To study the effects of ice cold water in a balloon in the small intestine in animals "to stun the absorbtive villi" to temporarily decrease fat asorbtion. ("gut reaction")

References & For Further Reading:

1. THE AMERICAN HEART ASSOCIATION - ABSTRACTS OF THIS 1996 ANNUAL MEETING IN NEW ORLEANS, LA.

2. THE AMERICAN HEART ASSOCIATION ABSTRACTS OF THE 1997 ANNUAL MEETING IN ORLANDO, FL. (SUPPLEMENT TO CIRCULATION OCT. 21, 1997.)

3. JOURNAL OF AMERICAN MEDICAL ASSOCIATION 1975-1998.

4. BRITISH MEDICAL JOURNAL 1975-1998.

5. JOURNAL OF ARTERIOSCLEROSIS, THROMBOSIS AND VASCULAR BIOLOGY.

6. THE AMERICAN JOURNAL OF CARDIOLOGY 1996-1998.

7. THE CANADIAN JOURNAL OF CARDIOLOGY JUNE, 1997. ABSTRACTS ON THE INTERNATIONAL CONFERENCE ON PREVENTIVE CARDIOLOGY IN MONTREAL, CANADA.

8. CARDIOLOGY CLINICS - 1980-1998. ESPECIALLY IMPORTANT - CARDIOLOGY CLINICS - FEBRUARY, 1996 - "CHANGING THE NATURAL HISTORY OF CORONARY ARTERY DISEASE - RISK FACTORS AND THEIR MODIFICATION (ISSN 0733-8651)

9. AMERICAN JOURNAL OF CLINICAL NUTRITION 1997-1998.

10. NEW ENGLAND JOURNAL OF MEDICINE - 1975-1998.

11. LANCET - 1975-1998.

12. JOURNAL OF ATHEROSCLEROSIS.

13. ATHEROSCLEROSIS RESEARCH

14. ANGIOLOGY

15. ARTERY.

16. LIPIDS AND LIPOPROTEINS - CURRENT PERSPECTIVES: D. JOHN BUTTERIDGE

17. FACTS AND FIGURES AMERICAN CANCER SOCIETY - 1997

18. SYNDROMES OF ATHEROSCLEROSIS: CORRELATION OF CLINICAL IMAGING FOR PATHOLOGY; VALENTIN FUSTER, M.D., PH.D. (ISBN - 087993-638-X)

19. CARDIOLOGY 1996 (THE BOOK NOT THE JOURNAL) ISBN - 0-87993-643-6; ISSN - 0275-0066

20. CARDIOLOGY 1997 (THE BOOK NOT THE JOURNAL) ISBN - 0-87993-677-0

21. HEART DISEASE - A TEXTBOOK OF CARDIOVASCULAR MEDICINE; EUGENE BRAUNWALD, M.D.: FIFTH EDITION.

22. THE HEART - (PREVIOUS EDITIONS BY J. WILLIS HURST, M.D.) 9TH EDITION R.W. ALEXANDER AND ROBERT C. SCHLANT, M.D. AND VALENTIN FUSTER, M.D. PH.D.

23. CLINICAL CARDIOLOGY - 6TH EDITION 1993; DR. SOKOLOW

24. THE PHARMACOLOGICAL BASIS OF THERAPEUTICS - NINTH EDITION; GOODMAN AND GILMAN

25. HARVARD HEART LETTER

26. JOURNAL WATCH CARDIOLOGY

27. CARDIOLOGY REVIEW

28. CARDIOLOGY TODAY

29. HEALTH NEWS - STRAIGHT TALK ON MEDICAL HEADLINES FROM THE PUBLISHERS OF NEW ENGLAND JOURNAL OF MEDICINE.

30. HARVARD WOMEN'S HEALTH WATCH

31. HARVARD MEN'S HEALTH WATCH

32. TUFTS UNIVERSITY HEALTH AND NUTRITION LETTER

33. JOHNS HOPKINS WHITE PAPERS, 1998.

34. JOHNS HOPKINS MEDICAL NEWSLETTER - HEALTH AFTER 50.

35. U.C. BERKELEY MEDICAL NEWSLETTER

36. MAYO CLINIC TELECONFERENCE ON PREVENTION OF ATHEROSCLEROSIS 1998.

37. ENVIRONMENTAL NUTRITION

36. NUTRITION ACTION HEALTH LETTER (FROM CENTER FOR SCIENCE IN PUBLIC INTEREST)

38. CANCER SMART

39. PRESCRIBERS NEWSLETTER

40. DEAN ORNISH'S PROGRAM FOR REVERSING HEART DISEASE; DR. DEAN ORNISH

41. THE PEOPLES GUIDE TO DEADLY DRUG INTERACTIONS-JOE GRAEDON AND TERESA GRAEDON, PH.D.

42. THE LIVING HEART-DR. MICHAEL DEBAKEY AND DR. ANTONIO GOTTO

43. REVERSING HEART DISEASE – JULIAN M. WHITAKER

44. CLINICAL SYMPOSIA: LIPID ABNORMALITIES AND CORONARY HEART DISEASE, SCOTT M. GRUNDY, M.D., PH.D. VOLUME 49, NO. 4, 1997 (NOVARTIS)

45. CARDIOVASCULAR TRIALS REVIEW (2ND EDITION) (KLONGER AND BIRNBAUM)

46. ANNALS OF INTERNAL MEDICINE

47. CARDIOVASCULAR ANESTHESIA

48. INTERNATIONAL JOURNAL OF RADIATION ONCOLOGY, BIOLOGY AND PHYSICS

49. JOURNAL OF THE NATIONAL CANCER INSTITUTE

50. SCIENTIFIC AMERICAN

51. NATURE

52. SCIENCE (JOURNAL OF THE AMERICAN ASSOCIATION FOR THE ADVANCEMENT OF SCIENCE — A.A.A.S.)

53. CARDIOLOGY SECRETS BY O. V. ADAIR, M.D. AND E. P. HAVRANECK

54. PHYSICIANS WEEKLY

55. A.M.A. NEWS

56. U.S. NEWS AND WORLD REPORT

57. TIME

58. NEWSWEEK

59. HERBS FOR HEALTH

60. HEALTH

61. USA TODAY

62. THE NEW YORK TIMES

63. THE SUN (BALTIMORE)

64. THE PHILADELPHIA ENQUIRER

65. THE CENTRE DAILY TIMES

66. THE WASHINGTON POST

67. THE ATLANTA CONSTITUTION

68. THE COUNTY OBSERVER (JUNIATA & MIFFLIN PA.)

69. THE JUNIATA SENTINEL

70. THE LEWISTOWN SENTINEL
71. THE PITTSBURGH POST GAZETTE
72. THE PATRIOT (HARRISBURG)
73. CNN NEWS
74. HEADLINE NEWS
75. NBC DATELINE
76. GOOD MORNING AMERICA
77. LARRY KING LIVE
78. OPRAH WINFREY SHOW
79. CNN HEALTHWATCH
80. CNN NEWS FROM MEDICINE
81. CNN NEWSSTAND
82. READERS DIGEST August 98 for Vit E

COMMENT: Tons of papers and miles of video tape. -Dr. Pai

1. STATISTICS from: PA DEPT OF HEALTH

2. EVIDENCE FOR MORE BENEFITS OF CHOLESTEROL LOWERING DRUGS-Andrew A. Skolnick JAMA Oct. 1 1997; 278: 1053 © 1997 American Medical Association (A.M.A.)

3. FISH CONSUMPTION AND THE RISK OF SUDDEN CARDIAC DEATH - C. M. Albert et al JAMA Jan 7 1998; 279: 23-28 © 1998 A.M.A.

4. CIGARETTE SMOKING AND PROGRESSION OF ATHEROSCLEROSIS. THE ATHEROSCLEROSIS RISK IN COMMUNITIES (ARIC) Study G Howard et al JAMA Jan 16 1998; 279: 119-124 © 1998 A.M.A.

5. MENTAL STRESS INDUCED MYOCARDIAL ISCHEMIA AND CARDIAC EVENTS W. Jiang et al JAMA June 5 1996; 275: 1651-1656 © 1996 A.M.A.

6. SLEEPINESS, DRIVING AND MOTOR VEHICLE CRASHES - James M Lyznicki, M.S.; M.P.H. June 17 1998; 279: 1908-1913 © 1998 A.M.A.

7. INCIDENCE OF ADVERSE DRUG REACTIONS IN HOSPITALIZED PATIENTS A META ANALYSIS OF PROSPECTIVE STUDIES J. Lazarou JAMA April 15 1998; 279: 1200-1205 © 1998 A.M.A.

8. EFFECTS OF RALOXIFENE ON SERUM LIPIDS AND COAGULATION FACTORS IN HEALTHY POSTMENO-

PAUSAL WOMEN B. W. Walsh et al JAMA May 13 1998; 279: 1445-1451 © 1998 A.M.A.

9. EFFECT OF GARLIC OIL PREPARATION ON SERUM LIPOPROTEINS AND CHOLESTEROL METABOLISM: A RANDOMIZED CONTROLLED TRIAL H. K. Berthold et al JAMA June 17 1998: 279:1900-1902 © 1998 A.M.A.

10. CIGARETTE SMOKING AND HEARING LOSS K.J. Cruickshanks et al JAMA June 3 1998:279:1715-1719 © 1998 A.M.A.

11. RANDOMIZED TRIAL OF ESTROGEN PLUS PROGRESTION FOR SECONDARY PREVENTION OF CORONARY HEART DISEASE IN POST MENOPAUSAL Women S. Hulley et al JAMA Aug 19 1998; 280: 605-613 © 1998 JAMA.

12. EFFECT OF LOCAL MEDICAL OPINION LEADERS ON QUALITY OF CARE OF ACUTE MYOCARDIAL INFARCTION: A RANDOMIZED CONTROL TRIAL S. B. Soumerai et al JAMA May 6 1998: 279: 1358-1363 © 1998 A.M.A.

13. PRIMARY PREVENTION OF ACUTE CORONARY EVENTS WITH LOVASTATIN IN MEN AND WOMEN WITH AVERAGE CHOLESTEROL LEVELS RESULTS OF AFCAPS/TEXCAPS J. R. Downs et al JAMA May 27 1998; 279: 1615-1622 © 1998 A.M.A.

14. ANTIATHEROTHROMBOTIC PROPERTIES OF STATINS IMPLICATION OF CARDIOVASCULAR EVENTS REDUCTION Robert S. Rosenson et al JAMA May 27 1998; 279: 1643-1650 © 1998 A.M.A.

15. COMMENTARY: LIPID LOWERING THERAPY IN LOW RISK PATIENTS Dr. Thomas A. Pearson M.D., Ph.D. JAMA May 27 1998; 279: 1659-1660 © 1998 A.M.A.

16. FISH CONSUMPTION AND SUDDEN CARDIAC DEATH - Editorial Dan Kromhout, Ph.D., M.P.H. JAMA Jan 7 1998; 279: 65 © 1998 A.M.A.

17. INTERFERENCE WITH CARDIAC PACEMAKERS BY CELLULAR TELEPHONES David L. Hayes et al New England Journal of Medicine May 22 1997; 336: 1473-1479 © 1997 Massachusetts Medical Society.

18. CORONARY RISK FACTORS AND PLAQUE MORPHOLOGY IN MEN WITH CORONARY DISEASE WHO

DIED SUDDENLY A. P. Burke et al N.E.J.M. May 1 1997; 336: 1276-1282 © 1997 Mass. Med. Soc.

19. THE COMPOSITION OF CORONARY ARTERY PLAQUES M.J. Davies N.E.J.M. May 1 1997; 336: 1312-1314 © 1997 Mass Med. Soc.

20. INFLAMMATION, ASPIRIN AND THE RISK OF CARDIOVASCULAR DISEASE IN APPARENTLY HEALTHY MEN P. M. Ridker et al N.E.J.M. April 3 1997; 336: 973-979 © 1997 Mass. Med. Soc.

21. INFLAMMATION, ATHEROSCLEROSIS, AND ISCHEMIC EVENTS EXPLORING THE HIDDEN SIDE OF THE MOON A. Maseri N.E.J.M. April 3 1997; 336: 1014-1016 © 1997 Mass. Med. Soc.

22. CAROTID ARTERY DISSECTION AFTER A PROLONGED TELEPHONE CALL Jean Jacques Mourad, M.D. NEJM Feb 13 1997; 336: 516 © 1997 Mass. Med. Soc.

23. EMERGENCY ROOM TRIAGE OF PATIENTS WITH ACUTE CHEST PAIN BY MEANS OF RAPID TESTING FOR CARDIAC TROPONIN I OR TROPONIN I, C. W. Hamm et al N.E.J.M. Dec 4 1997; 337:1648-1653 © 1997 Mass. Med. Soc.

24. HARDENED FAT, HARDENED ARTERIES Editorial Tim Byers N.E.J.M. Nov. 20 1997; 337: 1544-1545 © 1997 Mass. Med. Soc.

25. PLATELET GLYCOPROTEIN IIB/IIIA RECEPTOR BLOCKADE IN UNSTABLE CORONARY DISEASE James H. Chesebro M.D. et al May 21 1998; 338: 1539-1541 © 1998 Mass. Med. Soc.

26. PROBUCOL AND MULTIVITAMINS IN THE PREVENTION OF RESTENOSIS AFTER CARDIAC ANGIOPLASTY J. C. Tardif et al NEJM Aug 7 1997; 337: 365-372 © 1997 Mass. Med. Soc.

27. ANTIOXIDANTS AND ATHEROSCLEROTIC HEART DISEASE Mario N. Diaz et al N.E.J.M. Aug 7 1997; 337: 408-416 © 1997 Mass. Med. Soc.

28. VALVULAR HEART DISEASE ASSOCIATED WITH FENFLURAMINE PHENTERAMINE H. M. Connolly et al N.E.J.M Aug 28 1997; 337: 581-558 © 1997 Mass. Med. Soc.

29. THE SLEEP OF LONG HAUL TRUCK DRIVERS Merril Mitler et al N.E.J.M. Sept 11 1997; 337: 755-761

30. PERNICIOUS ANEMIA CORRESPONDENCE Oren Zimhony N.E.J.M. April 2 1998; 338: 995 © 1998 Mass. Med. Soc.

31. HYPERHOMOCYSTEINEMIA AS A RISK FACTOR FOR DEEP VEIN THROMBOSIS CORRESPONDENCE by Marco Cattaneo M.D. et al N.E.J.M. Sep 26 1996; 335: 974-976 © 1996 Mass. Med. Soc.

32. EFFECTS OF HORMONE REPLACEMENT THERAPY ON FIBRINOLYSIS IN POST MENOPAUSAL WOMEN S. E. Gabriel et al N.E.J.M. March 6 1997; 336: 683-689 © 1997 Mass. Med. Soc.

33. WORKING HOURS AS A RISK FACTOR FOR ACUTE MYOCARDIAL INFRACTION IN JAPAN: CASE CONTROL STUDY Shigeru Sokejima et al BMJ Sept 19 1998; 317: 775-780 © 1998 British Medical Journal (BMJ)

34. CHOLESTEROL: HOW LOW IS LOW ENOUGH? REACHING TARGET LEVELS MAY BE BETTER THAN RELATIVE REDUCTIONS A. Rosengren BMJ August 15 1998; 317: 425-426 © 1998 BMJ

35. THE END OF TRIGLYCERIDES IN CARDIOVASCULAR RISK ASSESSMENT? RUMOURS OF DEATH ARE GREATLY EXAGGERATED Naveed Satar, Chris J Packard and John R Petrie BMJ August 29 1998; 317: 553-554 © 1998 BMJ

36. ALCOHOL AND CANCER Editorial Svend Sabroe BMJ Sept 26 1998; 317: 827 © 1998 BMJ

37. POPULATION BASED COHORT STUDY OF THE ASSOCIATION BETWEEN ALCOHOL INTAKE AND CANCER OF THE UPPER DIGESTIVE TRACT Morten Gronbaek et al BMJ Sept 26 1998; 317: 844-848 © 1998 BMJ

38. WHY WINE MIGHT BE LESS HARMFUL THAN BEER AND SPIRITS Science Commentary Abi Berger, Science Editor BMJ Sept 26 1998; 317: 848 © 1998 BMJ

39. SCANDINAVIAN SIMVASTATIN SURVIVAL STUDY LANCET 1994; 344: 1383-1389 © 1994 LANCET

40. PREVENTION OF CORONARY HEART DISEASE WITH PRAVASTATIN IN MEN WITH HYPERCHOLESTEROLEMIA THE WEST OF SCOTLAND CORONARY PREVENTION Study Shepherd J. et al NEJM 1995; 333: 1301-1307 © 1995 Mass. Med. Soc.

41. LIPOPROTEIN AND CORONARY ATHEROSCLEROSIS STUDY Am J Cardiology 1997: 80: 278-286 © 1997 Am J. of Cardiology

42. DESIGN AND RATIONALE OF THE AIRFORCE/TEXAS CORONARY ATHEROSCLEROSIS PREVENTION STUDY (AFCAPS/TEXCAPS) AM J Cardiol 1997; 80: 287-293 © 1997 Am J Cardiol

43. RELATION BETWEEN IRON STORES AND NON-INSULIN DEPENDENT DIABETES IN MEN: CASE CONTROL STUDY. Jukka T. Salonen et al from Finland BMJ 1998; 317: 7 © 1998 BMJ

A question frequently asked to me is what does a plaque feel like? Coronary plaques are very small but the carotid plaques removed during an operation feel like a gummy candy with a hard stone inside.

AFTER READING THE BOOK YOU GET THE FOLLOWING IMPRESSION

1 **We have a very high rate of cardiovascular disease.**

2 We do not get enough sleep.

3 We live a very sedentary life.

4 A **big** segment of the American population is **overweight or obese.**

5 If we do not sleep and are sedentary what exactly are we doing?

6 We get prescriptions which we do not fill and do not take the medications as we are supposed to.

7 Ever since the criteria for ideal weight changed to a lower number, overnight a large segment of the newly overweight population claim that they have heavy bones or a heavy musculature or a large frame.

CAFÉ OF THE FUTURE Waiter to Customer: "Sir, could I bring your Folic Acid, B6, B12, Vitamin C, and Vitamin E with your red wine and green tea [two hours] before your tuna steak?"

124

ABOUT THIS BOOK

Text, research compiled by: Dr. Narendra Pai. Illustrations by Dr. Narendra Pai -computer enhanced by Big Air Graphics www.bigairphoto.com

TO ORDER THIS BOOK

For 1-10 copies send check or money order, $23.98 + $4.02 shipping and handling for each copy

To: **Stop Heart Disease Now!**
P.O. Box 787
Lewistown, PA 17044-0787

Allow 4 to 6 weeks for delivery. For faster service send money order for $23.98 and $7.02 for shipping and handling.
International orders - $23.98 + $14.02 shipping and handling. (money orders in U.S. funds)
For orders more than 10 books, Fax order to 717-248-0717.

Soon available on the internet at:

www.drusa.com

(PA residents add 6% tax to the value of the book and shipping and handling)
Shipping rates are subject to change without notice.

DISCLAIMERS:

1. The opinions in this book are solely of the author's and not of the Lewistown Hospital or its medical staff.

2. **Do not self treat - consult your doctor before starting or stopping any treatment.**

3. **Most of the drugs mentioned in this book are not recommended for pregnant women, potentially pregnant women or growing children.**

4. **The only thing permanent about medical knowledge is that it changes constantly. So keep informed and discuss any new knowledge of the disease or the drugs with your doctor.**

Corrections: Page 58, pt 116. Non-sexual chlamydia (Pneumoniae) does cause heart disease.

Additions:

1. Framingham study data shows that **elevated systolic blood pressure as the best predictor of cardiovascular morbidity and mortality.**

COMMENT: **Most physicians ignore** elevated isolated systolic BP and pay more attention to elevated diastolic BP.

2. Overwork or underwork increases heart disease risk. (BMJ Sept 19 1998; 317:775-780)

3. Through any type of alcohol is a strong risk factor for upper digestive cancer, resveratrol a substance in grapes and wine has been shown to **inhibit the initiation, promotion and progression of cancer** (prevent cancer) whereas **beer of spirits** **promote cancer.** Alcohol blocks the metabolism of nitrosamines so they enter the circulation and enter other organs where they are activated to carcinogens. BMJ Sept 26 1998; 317: 827, 844-848.

COMMENT: Wine is fine, avoid evil spirits. Drink wine with fresh grape juice, fresh blueberry juice and other fresh fruits (Remember the Lyon Study Mediterranean Diet reduces cardiovascular and cancer risk) Avoid spirits and beer with well done meat, bacon, nitrites and don't smoke.

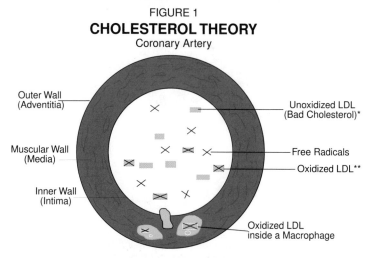

FIGURE 1
CHOLESTEROL THEORY
Coronary Artery

Outer Wall
(Adventitia)

Unoxidized LDL
(Bad Cholesterol)*

Free Radicals

Oxidized LDL**

Muscular Wall
(Media)

Inner Wall
(Intima)

Oxidized LDL
inside a Macrophage

* Unoxidized LDL, or "Bad Cholesterol", can be decreased by Cholesterol-lowering drugs.
**Oxidation of LDL can be minimized by Vitamin E and other antioxidants

Copyright © 1998 Dr. Pai

FIGURE 2
CHOLESTEROL THEORY
Coronary Plaque Formation

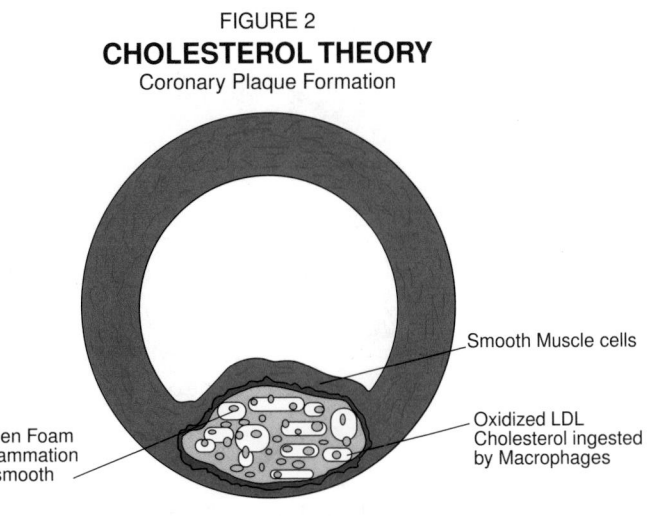

Smooth Muscle cells

Cholesterol-laden Foam cells cause inflammation and growth of smooth muscle cells

Oxidized LDL Cholesterol ingested by Macrophages

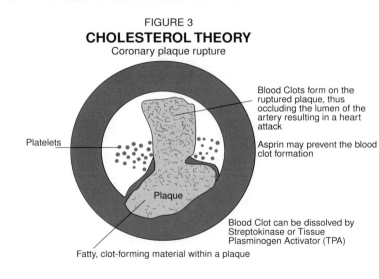

FIGURE 3
CHOLESTEROL THEORY
Coronary plaque rupture

Platelets

Plaque

Blood Clots form on the ruptured plaque, thus occluding the lumen of the artery resulting in a heart attack

Asprin may prevent the blood clot formation

Blood Clot can be dissolved by Streptokinase or Tissue Plasminogen Activator (TPA)

Fatty, clot-forming material within a plaque

129

FIGURE 4
HOMOCYSTEINE THEORY
Coronary Artery

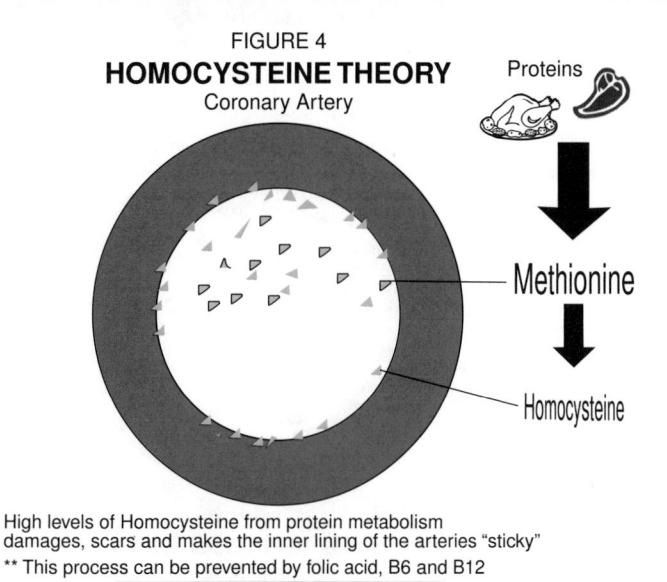

Proteins

Methionine

Homocysteine

High levels of Homocysteine from protein metabolism
damages, scars and makes the inner lining of the arteries "sticky"

** This process can be prevented by folic acid, B6 and B12

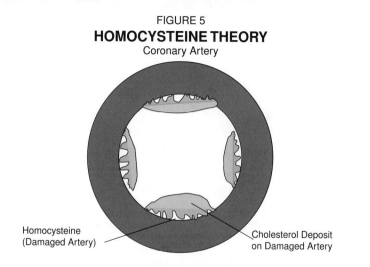

FIGURE 5
HOMOCYSTEINE THEORY
Coronary Artery

Homocysteine
(Damaged Artery)

Cholesterol Deposit
on Damaged Artery

131

FIGURE 6
CORONARY ARTERY
Stable Plaque

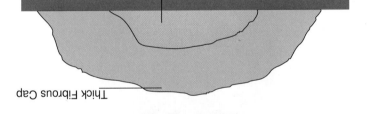

Thick Fibrous Cap

Small Lipid Core

132

FIGURE 7
CORONARY ARTERY
Unstable Plaque

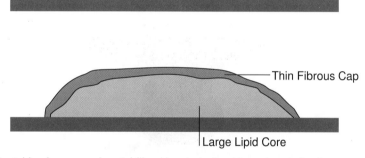

Thin Fibrous Cap

Large Lipid Core

Unstable plaque can be stabilized by cholesterol lowering statin drugs

FIGURE 8
CORONARY ARTERY
Plaque Rupture

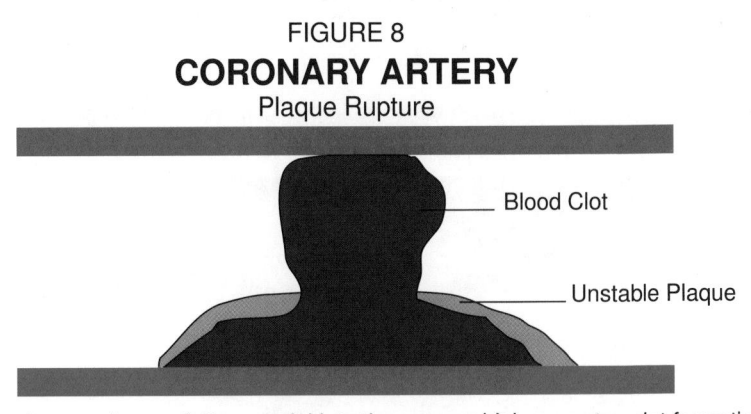

— Blood Clot

— Unstable Plaque

Unstable plaque releases fatty material into the artery which promotes clot formation

134